I0260807

HOW TO Reset Reframe AND Reshape

HOW TO Reset Reframe AND Reshape

A MOTHER'S GUIDE TO CHANGING HER MINDSET ABOUT FITNESS AND HER BODY

CASSIE MORELL

Founder of the **ReShapeHER** Program

How to Reset, Reframe, and Reshape:
A Mother's Guide to Changing Her Mindset About Fitness and Her Body

www.CassieMorell.com

Disclaimer: Please note that all information in this book is provided for educational purposes only and should not replace medical and/or psychiatric advice. The use of this book implies your acceptance of this disclaimer.

First edition 2024

Printed in the USA

ISBN 979-8-9909318-0-0 (Hard Cover)

ISBN 979-8-9909318-1-7 (Paperback)

ISBN 979-8-9909318-2-4 (eBook)

Library of Congress Control Number: 2024913145

Editing by Kevin Anderson & Associates, www.ka-writing.com

Photography by Melissa Jones, 3816 Creative, www.3816creative.com

Video production by Gary Sarcione, Stream of Vision Productions

Cover and interior formatting by Becky's Graphic Design®, LLC

www.BeckysGraphicDesign.com

Publisher's Cataloging-in-Publication Data

Names: Morell, Cassie, author.

Title: How to reset , reframe , and reshape : a mother's guide to changing her mindset about fitness and her body / Cassie Morell.

Description: Includes bibliographical references. | Cassie Morell, 2024.

Identifiers: LCCN: 2024913145 | ISBN: 979-8-9909318-0-0 (hardcover) | 979-8-9909318-1-7 (paperback) | 979-8-9909318-2-4 (ebook)

Subjects: LCSH Postnatal care. | Physical fitness for women. | Exercise for women. | Mothers--Health and hygiene. | BISAC HEALTH & FITNESS / Women's Health

Classification: LCC RG801 .M67 2024 | DDC 613.7/045--dc23

CASSIE MORELL

Contents

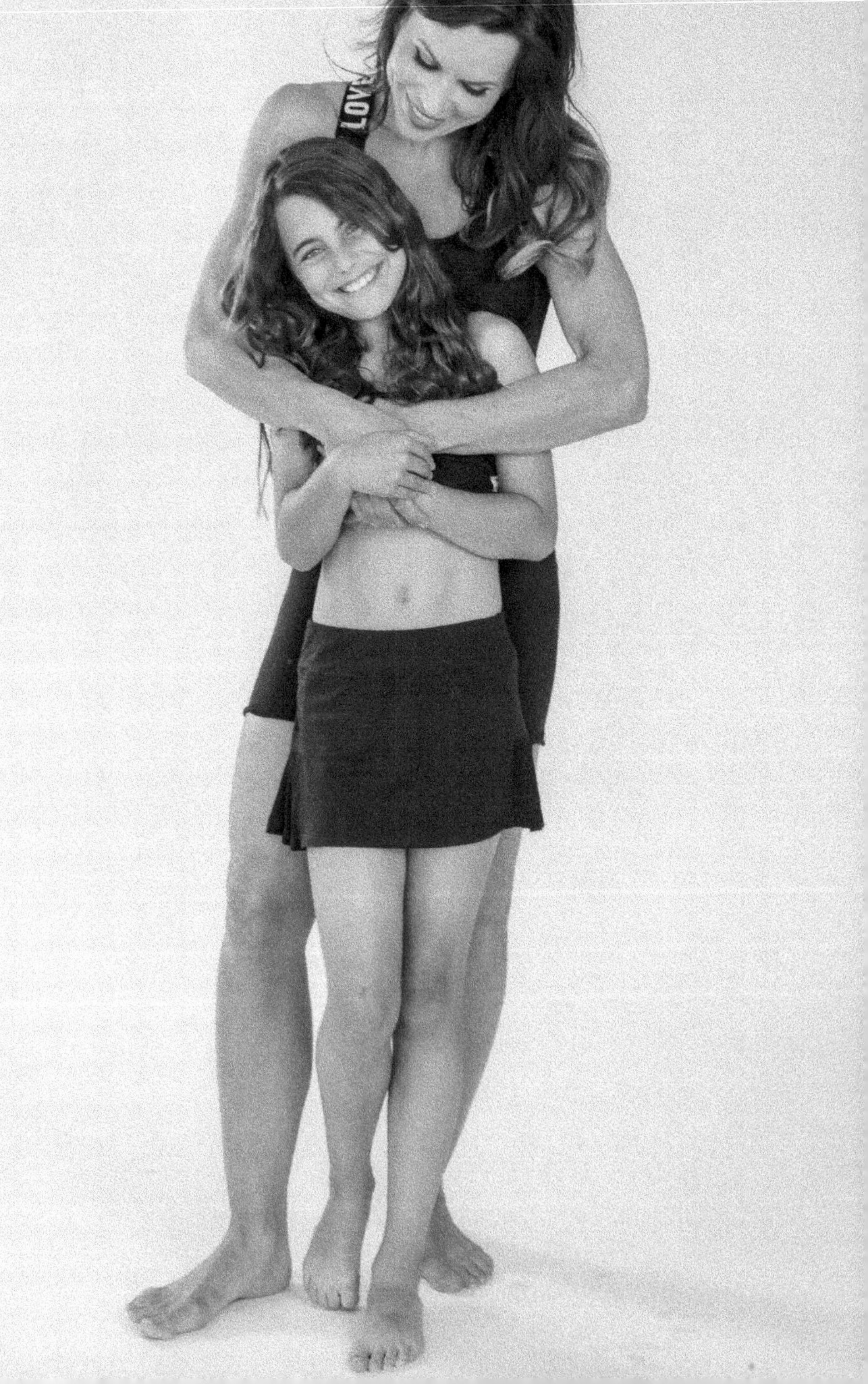

Dedication

MY DEAR, SWEET CATALINA,

This book is my dedication to you. Every thought, word, and page was fueled by my intent to ensure that you are able to embrace motherhood in your future, without the fear of losing yourself physically. My hope is that by reading this book, you will be able to enjoy all of the precious moments that being a mother has to offer, without hearing a voice of doubt fill your mind when it comes to regaining your fitness. This book is a representation of my healing journey as a mother. . . the part of me that refuses to carry the dysfunctions of the past, fighting hard to break crippling cycles that are based solely on a lack of education and a foundation of insecurity. This journey would never have been traveled had it not been for you. . . my firstborn.

Each chapter of this book represents a healing process that I am so grateful I can pass on to you. As you read my words, you can understand the importance of self-love. You can appreciate that aesthetics isn't all that defines our state of health. Although it is natural to compare ourselves to others, you can read my life's lessons on why comparison is futile and why we only have ourselves to blame if we continue this process. You will understand that even our health system may not support the education we need when it comes to achieving optimal health. You will become better at identifying the pitfalls that mothers fall prey to, and know how to avoid them by practicing the techniques I discuss in this book. Ultimately, you will learn how to take control of your nutrition and fitness, lending you to live a healthy life and passing on these valuable lessons to your family.

Through this book, Catalina, you will one day be a beacon of light for other mothers, helping them see how they can be the best version of themselves. I find incredible joy in knowing that you will be able to impart the same knowledge to them with an incredible amount of confidence, as you've been able to witness the living results in your life. You will know what it means to "trust the process," giving yourself grace and accepting whatever season your body may be in. You will one day embody what it means to be a healthy, fit mom.

As your mom, I encourage you to take this knowledge but never stop learning! Keep evolving into the best version of who *you* are. Your food is your fuel, but so is your wisdom. Remember, you are never on a "diet" and you never define yourself by a number. Your mind is one of your greatest superpowers and the greatest of influences on your body. Fuel your mind with good thoughts, good education and good intentions. You can be whatever your mind thinks you can be.

Okay, Mom will step off her soapbox.

I love you forever and always, Catalina.

Mom xoxo

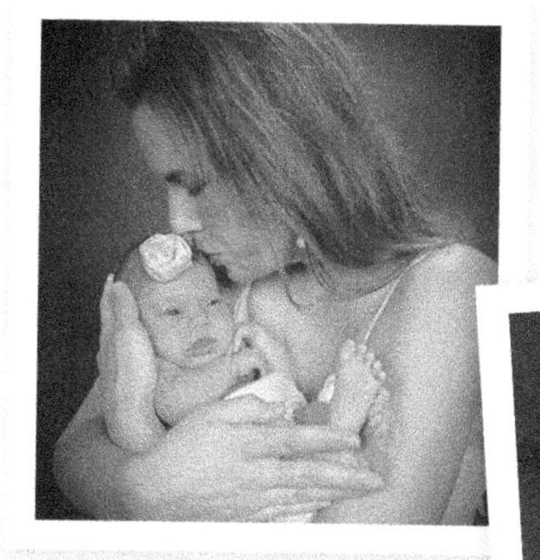
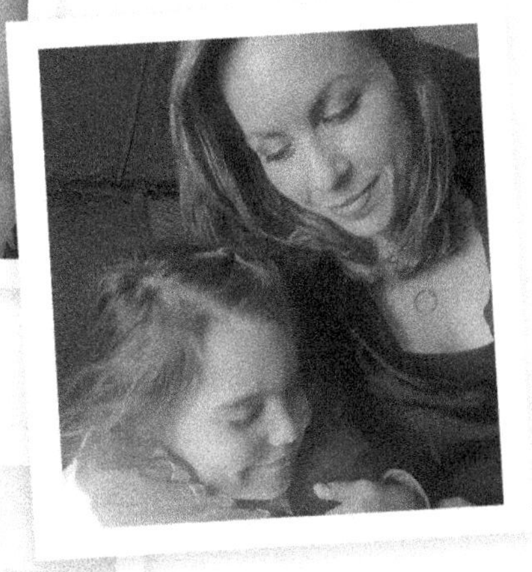
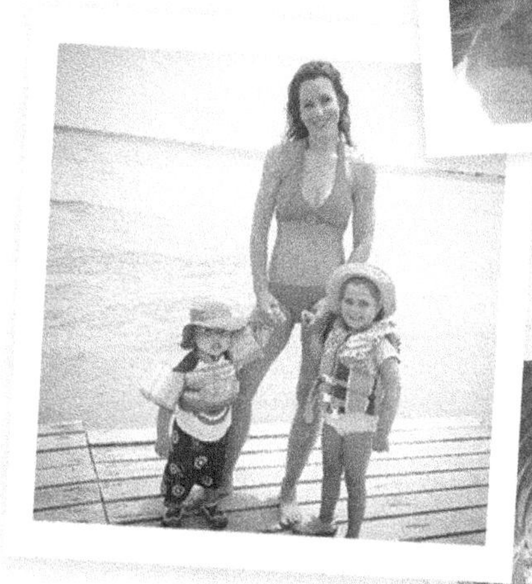
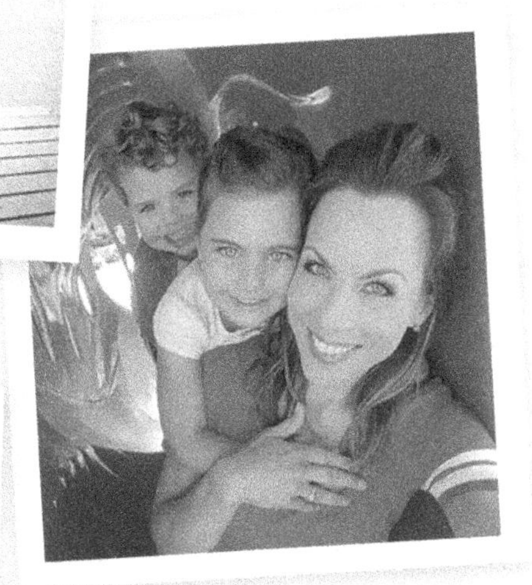
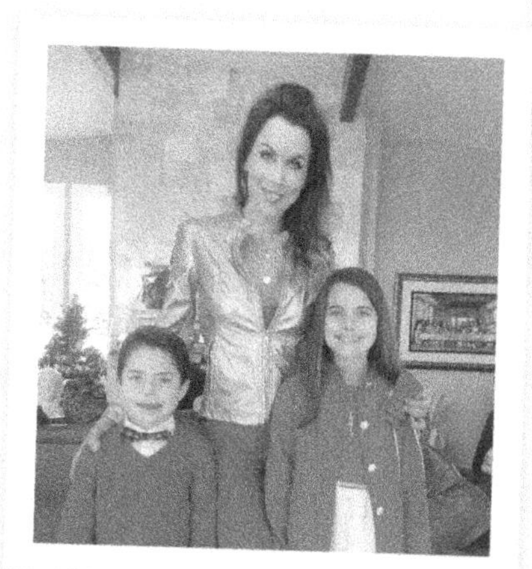

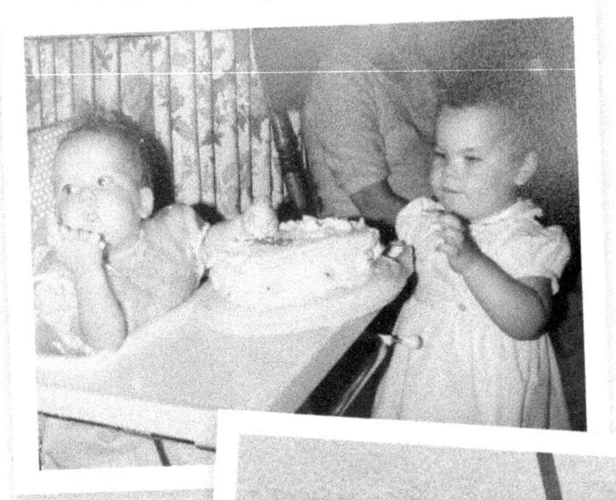

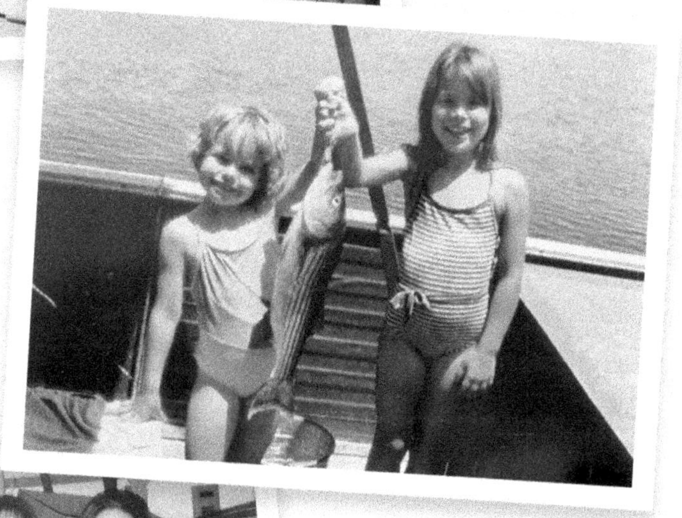

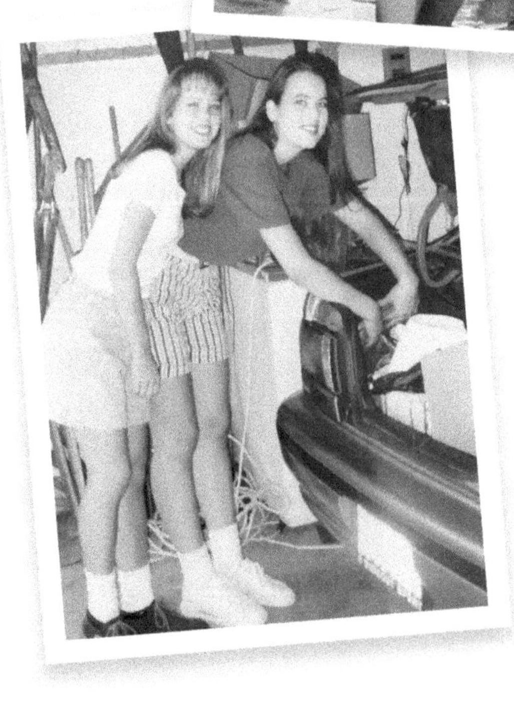

Introduction

AS ONE OF THREE GIRLS raised by a single mother, I saw her struggling to maintain her fitness with a busy schedule and little understanding of how to take care of her health. I have vivid memories of her running around in a pair of leotards and tights, doing aerobics, drinking Diet Coke, and eating her two plain rice cakes for lunch. She was always on a fad diet, kept the refrigerator packed with nonfat food items, and was constantly tied to her scale. Her self-worth was determined by the number that read on this scale and also the one that was sewn on the back of her jeans. She was often afraid to eat and had a horrible relationship with food. Her constant struggle with her self-worth, which was tied to her unhealthy fitness practices and supplements, negatively impacted her health and the mental health of my sisters and me. My middle sister and I have maintained a close relationship over the years (she's pictured with me below). We often talk about how difficult those younger years were for us. It is because of these personal experiences that I'm determined to not continue these dysfunctional patterns with my own daughter and work hard to be a better role model for her when it comes to health and fitness.

Unfortunately, I know many women whose mothers had the same practices of which they're replicating unknowingly, as they haven't had the time or resources to put toward a true understanding of fitness. Additionally, our society continues to breed this type of behavior in women. It's not just the supplement promotions that cause dependency and false promises, but also the fad workouts and diets that typically promote dramatic results that don't end up with long-term weight loss or health benefits. Sadly, social media has made it easier and more effective for these types of fads to be promoted, as they do this behind the picture of young fitness models whose unblemished bodies haven't experienced childbirth, nor have they experienced the stress and demands of being a busy mom.

With these unrealistic images, mothers eventually face a dead end in their thoughtful pursuit of having a better body composition, as they fall astray to these falsifications and end up buying into the concept that they are past the point of being able to achieve their fitness goals. Without the proper education surrounding fitness, they start to put the blame on aging and hormones. Ultimately, many moms give up on the idea that it's possible to have a sexy and healthy body after the child-bearing years altogether, and lose their motivation to pursue any form of fitness goals. They desperately need a **RESET** when it comes to their overall thought-process when it comes to fitness.

For many years, although growing up athletic, I fell into some of my mother's same detrimental fitness attempts. I struggled with my weight and did my fair share of crash dieting and cardio in order to achieve my aesthetic goals. My body, although athletic, was tired of unsuccessful attempts over the years, and at the ripe age of 18, I was diagnosed with hypothyroidism. This diagnosis seemed to make my fitness attempts all that more difficult to achieve. Later in my life, after having both of my kiddos and turning the age of 40, I decided to spend time trying to figure out if I could debunk the perpetual myth that it wasn't possible to have a better body at an older age and after the childbearing years. I committed to the process of developing my postpartum physique as I wanted to compete in bodybuilding. During this process of working on my body composition after having kids, I began to more thoroughly understand the pitfalls that women fall into (especially mothers) that derail their body composition goals. I learned how to successfully avoid these pitfalls with my own body to reach my fitness goals, (what I term the **REFRAME** period of my life). During this process, I began to realize that the answers to avoiding these pitfalls were often not shared by the fitness community, as they were coveted as "hooks" to keep clients, as many fitness gurus are coaches that promote societal "quick fixes" to profit their businesses. I started seeing how easy it becomes for many women (especially mothers) to end up in the snares of these bad coaches and practice these vicious cycles of unhealthy fitness practices, resulting in unmet fitness goals and eventually placing the blame on aging or hormones.

Once I was able to gain my own confidence in trusting the knowledge that I had learned in my own postpartum pursuit of fitness, I was able to steer away from my old ways and develop (**RESHAPE**) the body composition I always wanted. And here's the crazy thing... I did it in my 40s and even after having babies! It was at that point that I knew I was an honest testament to what worked. I felt empowered and knew I needed to put all of this valuable information about my fitness success into a single program and share it with all of my fellow mothers through a book, to empower them also. It was time for me to turn my motive into a reality, and so I began writing...

As a busy mother of two young kids, I know how time-consuming and expensive trying to achieve an education in fitness can be. This is why I was so compelled to share my fitness wisdom with mothers like you. Through my fitness journey, I've been able to create and fine-tune a solid fitness plan that combats all four of the pitfalls I discuss, which keep mothers from achieving their fitness goals. This program can be tailored to any busy mom regardless of where she practices her fitness and the amount of time she has to do so. My ReShapeHER program has led me to my own fitness success as well as with the many mothers I've had the pleasure to work with.

The ReShapeHER program can provide fitness clarity for any mother who dedicates her time to taking care of their family and has little time to invest in herself... especially in her fitness. Oftentimes, these unsung heroes are busy making sure their children are clothed and fed, hitting their milestones successfully, and living their best little lives, while they hope to have a successful shower and a good night's rest at the end of the day. The bodies of these heroes have contributed to the "miracle of life" and all of its stages, but these mothers may feel like they don't have fitness support when it comes to picking up the postpartum pieces, tackling the seasons that follow, as they work to achieve a better body composition postpartum.

Time that might have been typically spent rushing to the gym after work is now spent making dinner or picking up and dropping off kids at school or extracurricular activities. Even when the newborn or toddler stage has ended, the priorities of children and family always take precedence, leaving mothers with little time to figure out how to navigate fitness into their busy schedules. With the little amount of time they have, they are left to tackle the muddied waters of the fitness industry, which leaves them confused and discouraged.

Because of this, quick fixes that the fitness industry likes to serve up on a silver platter, which offer hollow promises through fad products and unrealistic timelines, become their source of fitness hope. The fitness industry is fully aware of this. It can be an expert at addressing fitness needs and filling them with shallow solutions.

With these unsuccessful solutions, it may leave a postpartum mother buying into the myth that reaching any pinnacle of great health at this stage of her life is simply not possible. The ReShapeHER program can give a mother like this the reins back when it comes to her fitness and her overall health. It can help her accomplish her fitness goals within a short period of time by helping her understand what she needs to do as it relates to her fitness practices.

Busy mothers are also easy prey for being caught in the snare of bad coaches because they know we have little time to dedicate to our fitness efforts. They take advantage of them as perpetual clients, by giving them only little bits of information over time, taking advantage of the one thing these mothers don't have. Most busy mothers may not have the resources to hire the best experts who can help them achieve the results they're looking for. And even if they do, many of these coaches aren't sharing fitness information with them, that empowers them and allows them to learn how to achieve their fitness goals on their own. Because of this, mothers become victims of failed fitness attempts and the frustrations of trying to figure out what works. They can become easily discouraged, internalizing some of the harmful and negative messages that society sends about the future of a woman's body after pregnancy and aging. Without fitness education and experience, these mothers often succumb to sadness and vulnerability when it comes to their fitness, paralyzing their abilities to achieve their optimal fitness health.

It is time to put an end to this vicious cycle! This can possibly happen with the education a postpartum mother can receive by reading this book and adopting the ReShapeHER program into her fitness journey, helping her reach her goals **in as little as 4-6 weeks!** *(Results vary based on individual responses.)*

I experienced ups and downs, pitfalls, and failures, when I began my postpartum fitness journey. However, these things all led me to the fitness success I've been able to achieve and share with you in this book. As you read through each page, you will be educated with a wealth of knowledge about fitness that will *save you both time and money* if you apply the principles of the ReShapeHER program in your fitness journey. I poured my valuable life experiences into this book in order to help you achieve the body of your dreams. It is my hope as a fellow mother that you take the pearls you learn from this book, apply them to your fitness, and also teach a fellow mother something, saving her both time and money in her fitness journey.

Fitness is a gift, and the knowledge that we obtain from it should be shared. It shouldn't be complicated or clouded with misinformation. Mothers, and women in general, should all be helping one another to achieve our fittest lives, contributing to an overall fit and healthy world not only for ourselves but also for our daughters. I know we can all agree that postpartum mothers in our world need more knowledge about fitness that saves them time and money in order for them to achieve better personal fitness. I hope we can one day achieve that. This book is my contribution.

As a mother of a beautiful daughter who will one day be a mother herself, it is my hope that by sharing my ReShapeHER program, her generation of postpartum mothers won't have to struggle with the unsuccessful attempts past generations have when it comes to achieving their fitness goals. It is my hope that this book is the start of a new wave of female empowerment, one that exploits the "smoke in mirrors" bullshit that has been spoon-feeding our past generations of mothers the fitness falsifications that have led them to failure in reaching their best body compositions and fitness goals. Enough is enough.

It is time for us to collectively raise the status of mothers through fitness education, awareness, and literacy. It is time for us to show ourselves, and our children, how to RESET our dysfunctional thought processes when it comes to fitness. It is time for us to REFRAME the way we think about what is possible when it comes to our fitness potential. And, it is time to optimally RESHAPE our bodies, by consistently practicing successful fitness habits that contribute to us reaching and maintaining our best overall health as moms. There's no better time than now.

Cassie

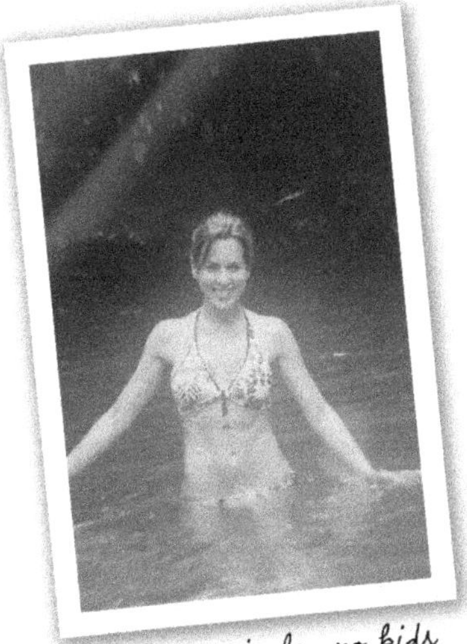

29 years, single, no kids

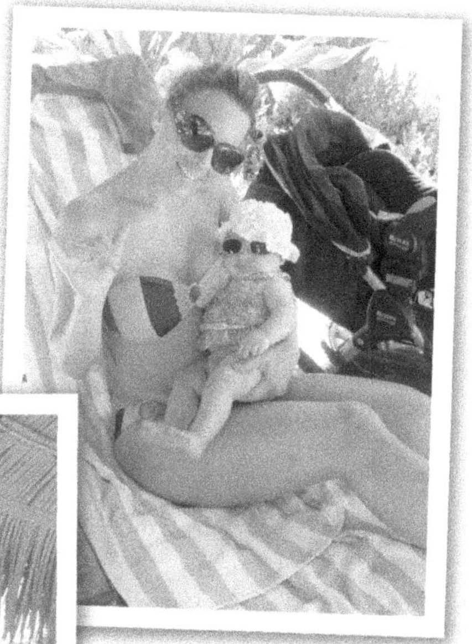

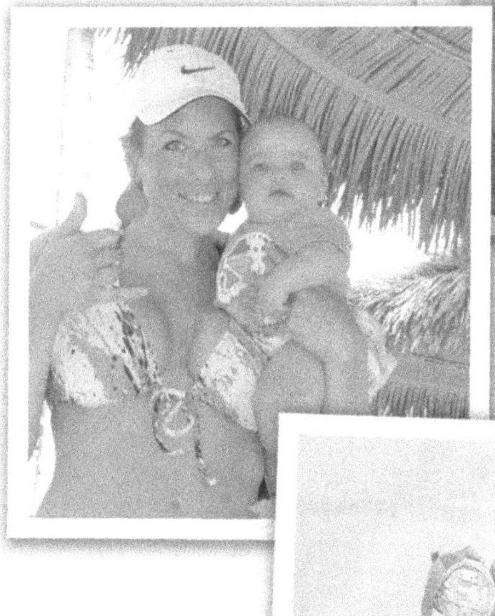

Post-baby body

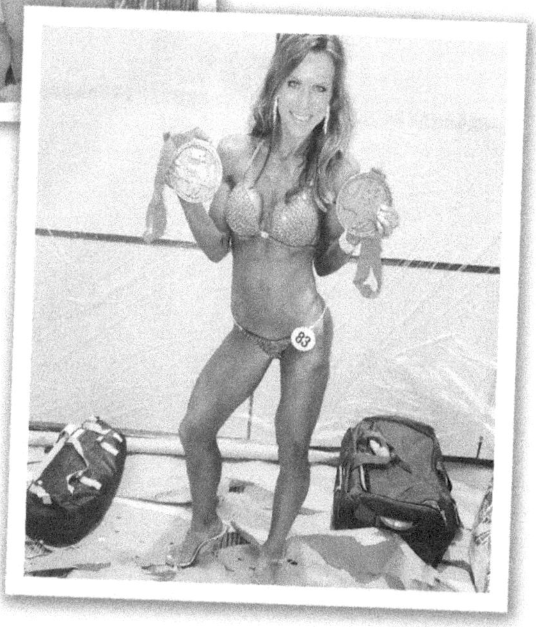

42 years old,
married,
mother of two

The RESET

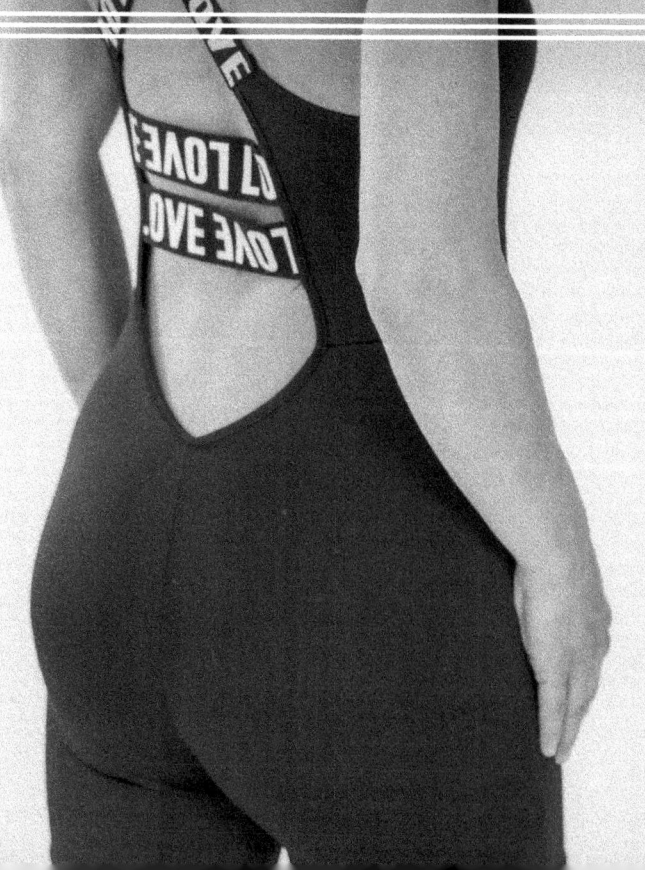

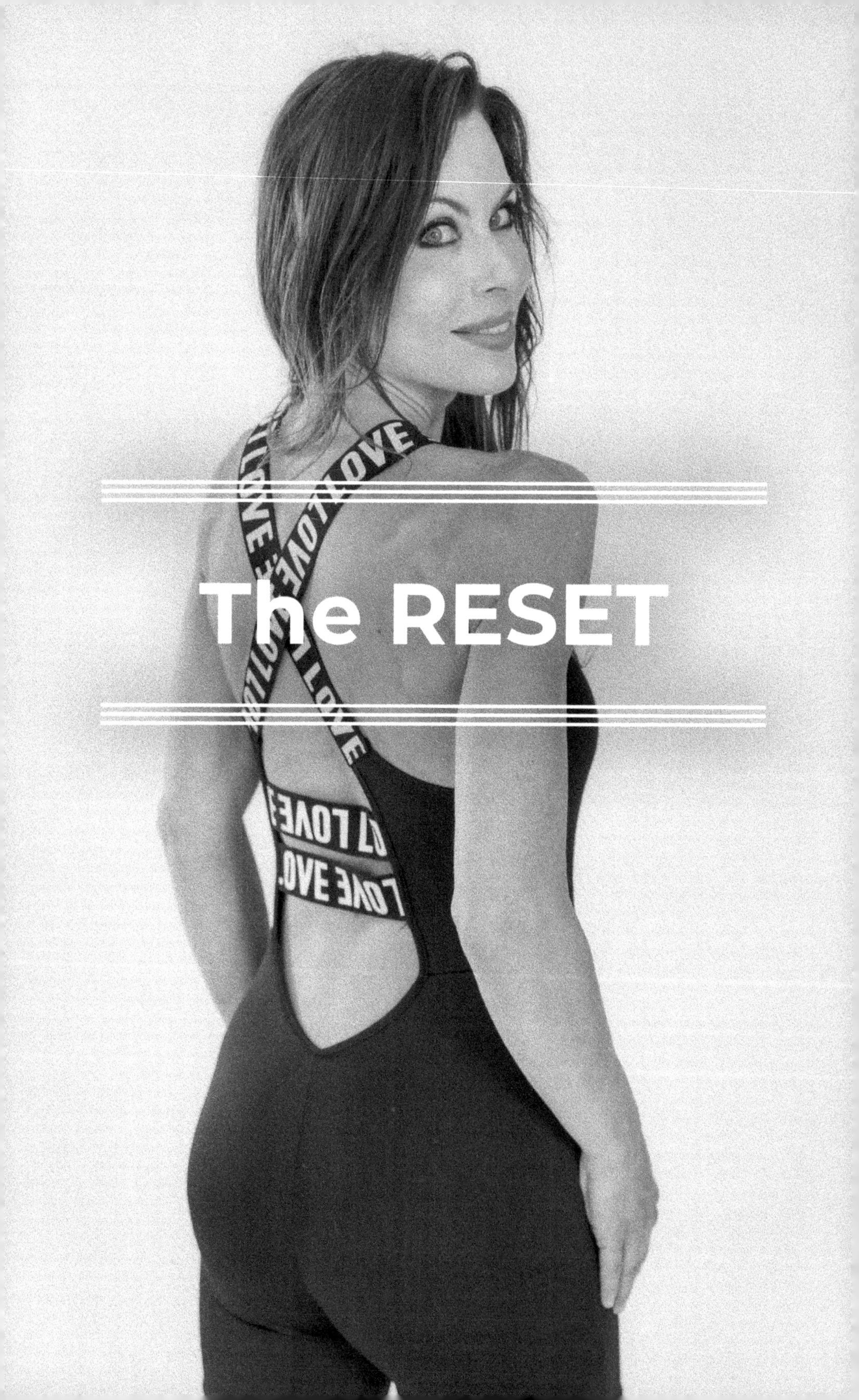

1

Fitness Success Starts with Self-Love

IT IS EASY IN THE age of the Social Media Revolution to develop ideal images of what female bodies should look like, based on the curated content of societal influencers. Images that are "easy on the eyes," radiant, and youthful sell... the aesthetics are what we see and the anticipated result of any type of product or program. The fitness industry is one that is largely focused on these aesthetics because it is assumed that if someone is healthy from the inside, their body will reflect that. The outward appearance is also what we are attracted to, with our natural senses. It's hard to take an industry like fitness and completely change it, but what we can do is identify its faults and do our best to make it more inclusive.

How we build on this inclusivity is through education. I've discussed my motivation for writing this book and how I hope to teach women (mothers specifically), about how they can achieve their fittest lives. This in turn will contribute to a healthy image of what fitness can look like for mothers and ultimately define their place in this Social Media Revolution.

As mothers, we have the power to create a movement that can ultimately redefine our place in the fitness world, and this all begins with how we identify with this place within ourselves. Do we believe as mothers that we have a place in this fitness space not only for ourselves but also for our daughters who might also be mothers? Are we tired of the curated images that society has plagued us with that portray the message that only women with no childbearing experience can achieve fitness success? These questions can all be answered confidently if we have a strong sense of self-love.

As mothers, we need to take responsibility to ensure that these curated images we're constantly being fed by society aren't what's defining our overall understanding of fitness. We have to be cautious, as it is easy to develop an over-fixation on the aesthetics of fitness, as we are a very visual society, and it can be easily assumed that our fitness aesthetics define our state of fitness health. We tend to forget that there are many other dimensions of health and fitness other than just the physical... there's also the mental and spiritual. As mothers, and females in general, we are taught from a very early age to compare ourselves. Perhaps this teaching stems from a history of being oppressed in a male dominated society, but it can damage our ability to strengthen our position in our society and keep us from reaching our gender goals. The act of comparison is what keeps us as women, from uniting and being more of an overall force in our world.

COMPARISON IS FUTILE

As a female and mother, I've experienced my fair share of comparison games. However, going through the process of bodybuilding in my 40s made me realize how destructive this game of comparison can be. As I graced the stage with women who had never experienced childbirth and whose bodies were young and tight, free from the scars of this experience, I was being judged on the same platform that they were. I almost became lost in my own insecurities as I had to learn to manage the disillusionment I was gaining from a sport that so heavily valued aesthetics. I had to trust myself and my abilities and carefully process my insecurities. I had to fight through the process of not allowing my jaded mindset to become my reality, derailing me from accomplishing my fitness goals.

I discuss further in this book why the act of comparison is futile when it comes to true body composition, but I also learned that it is futile when it comes to supporting any type of mental or spiritual health. It is a dirty game that devalues the significance of women and lessons our overall power in society.

This game of constant comparison is directly associated with our insecurities. We often get caught up with idealizing what others have that we may not, or feeling shame for carrying the scars of life experiences that should be deemed as a sign of heroism, but in lieu of this, it is thought of as a flaw. Oftentimes what makes the game of comparison so easy to play for many mothers is that their internal voice behind the insecurities can be loud. I know personally that the voice that screams my insecurities and doubts seems as if it's using a megaphone inside my head. She is the voice of all of my doubts, and sometimes her main goal is to stop me from believing I am capable of achieving that which I'm pursuing.

THE NEGATIVE "VOICE" OF DOUBT

Over the years I've learned to familiarize myself with this voice and today I deem "her" as nameless, other than an obnoxious bitch. While at first she gained my full attention, she will now scream to a mind that has learned to compartmentalize what she's saying and only react once her concerns have been rationalized. I've often wondered why this voice seems as though she can speak to me the way she does, and I can only hope that over time the volume will lessen as I've learned to handle it in the healthy way I've learned how. I'm not sure how I developed a voice that speaks this way to me about my insecurities (I'm assuming it stems from childhood trauma or my years of trying to be a perfectionist), but what I do know is that I can't let her derail me from achieving my goals. Regardless of what she has to say, she will learn that my practice of self-love will come before ridiculing myself over my insecurities and giving in to the game of comparison.

As wicked as it can be, there's a natural and unassuming aspect to the art of comparison. It is human nature to want to associate, relate, and feel part of something. Sharing commonalities with others is what draws us together, but not sharing these is also what sometimes tears us apart. The fitness industry can effectively bring out the commonalities of what people share but can also ostracize those who don't share them. It is an industry that has become very effective in glorifying the commonalities that reflect the pinnacle of health achievements but does little for those who may share a part of these or possibly none at all.

BODY SHAMING

Body shaming has become viral, as social media platforms make it even easier to communicate what these commonalities should look like and how they are viewed. This has bred the practice of criticism about bodies or physiques that don't reflect what are deemed as acceptable. This often discourages those who don't fit into the norm from pursuing their fitness ambitions, and can even result in them being mocked or criticized for not doing so. Body shaming has placed stigmas on particular body types and sizes. It has even discriminated against the most popular of celebrities and has become a big problem in our modern-day society. As mothers, we are unfortunately all partially to blame for the glorification of perfection and all that is intangible. We are the ones who continue to seek all of this instead of appreciating our unique differences. We often try to romanticize fitness, waiting for a potion or supplement to bring us those "feel-good" results, when in actuality we fail to accept the fact that the only way we can obtain these results is by putting in the work to achieve them. We create a world of sensory overload as we spend too much time looking at fitness models who are photoshopped and airbrushed. We allow filtered images to destroy our sense of normality as they cover the hard-earned stretch marks that are much more realistic. Unfortunately natural bodies and unfiltered images have lost their earned appreciation and respect.

With all of these unhealthy practices, we have become so sensitive with our unrealistic perceptions that we shelter ourselves from reality. We have ultimately created this environment where body shaming can flourish, as this intangible idea of perfection is what captivates our attention more than what is genuine and more relatable. As much as we may communicate how much we despise this phenomenon, we also feed into it. As much as we hate that we compare ourselves to these unrealistic images in our minds, we continue to compare ourselves to this false sense of reality.

PERFECTION DOESN'T EXIST

This intangible idea of perfection is also what separates us as mothers. We often buy into the idea that we have to "do it all" in order to be successful in our roles. If we can't work a job, be a sexy wife, keep a perfectly clean house, be a short-order cook, tend to all of the needs of our children, and be the best friend, we often think of ourselves as failing. When we fail at any of these things temporarily, we are riddled with guilt and feel the insecurity that comes along with it. What adds to the remorse are constant images of other mothers who are seemingly making this all possible through their highlight reels on social media.

What we fail to remember is that negative content (which is a part of life) is rarely posted on social media, but the positive images we see of others continue to drive our insecurities. What we fail to realize is that these positive posts are often made as a result of justifications for the insecurities of the women posting them. These insecurities that come from being connected on social media can also be the very things that drive us apart as women and mothers. Instead of building on our self-love, we practice self-criticism more often, blaming ourselves for everything we're not. We begin to tear ourselves down and allow these insecurities to overshadow the beautiful attributes we bring to this world, all stemming from what is essentially a facade and not a true reality.

This fairytale we buy into that is often portrayed, makes the entire process of motherhood a difficult one. As changes are endured through pregnancy, they are often welcomed with worry and the notion that if they become too great, a mother will lose her body entirely to the process. I distinctly remember worrying so much about the process of my body gaining weight to support my baby that my obstetrician had to write me a therapeutic note on her prescription pad. She told me to tape this note up on my mirror as my daily reminder that I would "love myself every day through my pregnancy and that I was beautiful no matter what my weight was on the scale."

It was incredibly difficult at times to remember to do this, especially when my body was going through changes that I couldn't control and made it difficult for me to see myself in the process. I was soon not able to see my toes when I looked down as my belly blocked my view. At one point, I swore my ass was a pillow as I sat down one day, as this area had managed to gain a large portion of my baby weight.

When I noticed other mothers experiencing pregnancy differently, whether they didn't have body image issues or just seemed to enjoy the uncontrollable process of their bodies changing, it made me angry and resentful. In order to understand any type of benchmark (especially with my first pregnancy), I began to compare myself to other women to try and understand how much these changes were affecting me and perhaps try and curb them if I felt like I wasn't making great progress in my pregnancy. I did this with no consideration of my uniqueness and not understanding that it was impossible to compare one mother to another. I knew better than this but the pressure I placed on myself was too great. I needed to practice more self-love during my pregnancies, although I found it very difficult at times.

As mothers we need to continue to remind ourselves that perfect doesn't exist! We need to stop the pursuit of perfection. In lieu of this idealism, we need to start chasing something that is the best version of us. If we want to be fit, we need to practice the best habits we know or learn and do them consistently. If we want to see results, we need to stop seeking these utopian images in our mind and replace them with kick-ass effort that results in individual transformation. The more we chase effort, humility, best practices, and shying away from comparing ourselves to others, the sooner we will start to see and appreciate individual results and not be let down by this unrealistic "perfect" we have a tendency to create in our minds.

This is why the best way to combat body shaming is through dropping this idea of perfect and practicing more self-love. That is, realize that the worst critics of our bodies can often be ourselves. For women especially, we get bogged down by trying to hit this arbitrary number on a scale or clothing size. Sadly, if we don't achieve these numbers, it can also affect our moods and our overall outlook on ourselves. I'll get into why scale weight is arbitrary later in this book, but the point is, we have to love ourselves a lot deeper than this. We can't define our abilities, progress, and overall worth down to a reading on a scale. We need to dig deeper and love ourselves on a much greater level.

SELF LOVE ISN'T SELFISH

When we learn to love ourselves on a deeper level, this allows us to not allow the setbacks to derail us as greatly. Although motivation won't always be there, on days we don't feel it, self-love can remind us why we are going through the actions anyway. Self-love will remind us of the priority that it is important to continue working on the best version of ourselves.

As mothers, we need to remember that self-love isn't selfish! We have to remember to not allow anyone to make us feel this way while we're practicing self-love. Self-love is loving one's own self to a healthy capacity. This allows us to love others to a greater level because our buckets are full. This is not the same as being selfish, as the secondary motive of practicing self-love is being one's best self so that we can, in turn, love others more. We can't be good mothers, wives, friends, or people unless we've taken the time to practice self-love. Without this practice, we become unhappy and possibly resentful or insecure. I'm sure we've all known "that mother" who lacks self-love... she's jealous, can't stop picking others apart, reflects her internal unhappiness. She may not be selfish by nature, but because she feels unloved by herself, she emulates this characteristic. By not practicing self-love, this mother's insecurity takes over and, ladies... insecurity is very *loud*!

Self-love is accepting yourself for who you are and the way you are. You don't have to be 100 percent happy with where you are, and you can strive to be better, but you love yourself on the journey. This love is your internal fuel. It is your support system when others are not or can't be. It is absolutely essential in order to be the best version of oneself. It isn't defined by a number, a look, a size, or an appearance. It is patient, kind, forgiving, and unconditional. It is the ultimate food for our souls.

Practicing self-love requires just that... practice. There are many times in life that you may find yourself realizing that you need to practice it more just like anything else. And just like many other things, the more you practice, the better you'll get. Even nature understands the importance of practicing self-love. I'm a big fan of orchids, and I have a collection of them in my bathroom. It was at the height of the COVID lockdown that I realized my orchids were blooming despite the pandemic that was going on. They were carrying on with their self-love journey and producing the most beautiful blooms I've seen since I owned them. I jotted down some simple "self-love" tips from them, as I enjoyed their beauty.

TIPS FOR SELF-LOVE

1. Learn to only require essentials... water, food, sunlight.
2. Exist to bring oxygen and joy to the world.
3. Despite any environmental tension, bloom predictably and eloquently in every season because that's what you're capable of
4. When a part of you stops the growth process, proceed to another.
5. Don't be frustrated with spending many months in a state of no bloom... your flowers will come in time and in season.

As mothers, we can be our own version of the orchid. We can be like a beautiful flower that doesn't need a constant reminder of its beauty, because deep down we know that if we're not in a state of bloom, it will come in due time. We can bring joy into our environments simply because we emulate it through this internal self-love. Our husbands, spouses, partners, children, and families will experience this joy and it will also positively affect them. Should our growth be stunted, we simply move on to another part of ourselves that we can grow successfully while continuing this process of self-love.

Learning to love yourself is so important in your fitness journey. The practice of self-love will lead to confidence and self-respect. This in turn will allow you to get the most out of your journey. Fitness itself is a form of self-love. It is taking the time out of the day for oneself, doing something that contributes to one's own self-care. It is knowing that although as a mother there's a busy day ahead, you'll be your "best self" by setting time aside to do what fuels your body. It can allow someone to reframe the way in which they view exercise and moving in general, making it a passion and not a chore. It is being present in whatever you're doing, allowing your body to speak to you if need be, and allowing yourself to listen. It is having respect for this voice and responding in the best way for you, not according to anyone else. It is the practice of telling yourself that YOU are important, YOU matter, and YOU are worthy.

YOUR SUPPORT SYSTEM

Along with finding the space for your practice of self love, it is critical that as a mother, you communicate the importance of this to your support system. By doing this, you allow others to understand how you value yourself and define healthy boundaries so you can successfully practice being the best version of YOU. Your support system can help you improve your overall health and can often provide you with mental, emotional and practical support when you may need it most. This system can hopefully be found at home, but can also be found outside the home in communities that share values that are in common with your own when it comes to health and fitness.

YOUR "WHY"

One of the most important reasons for practicing self-love in fitness is that it is required to establish and focus on your "WHY." Your "WHY" will serve as the glue for your motivation, especially on the days it's hard to find. (I will discuss how you will develop your "WHY" in the next chapter.) It will be the soul-gripping reason why you want to achieve your fitness goals in the first place. There will be many times along your fitness journey that you won't be motivated and your "WHY" will be the catapult to get you beyond this temporary feeling. Your "WHY" will ultimately define your willingness to continue on your fitness journey. Motivation, you'll learn, will be a fleeting feeling that is nice when it's experienced but isn't required to accomplish your goals. What will be required will be your discipline and a laser-focus on your "WHY."

Ultimately, with a strong sense of self-love, your vision ("WHY") will become clearer and you will become more willing to go out of your comfort zone to do the things that require you to be successful. When self-love is strong, it fuels your mind and this vision, allowing you to face your insecurities and all of those things that make you uncomfortable. You can begin to create boundaries for your insecurities and the fear of them will no longer be a setback in your life. You will be able to quiet that loud voice (if you have one) inside your head. Not every day will be easy, but with practice it will get easier.

Practicing self-love and developing a "WHY" that focuses us on our goals is an important practice that goes beyond the boundaries of just fitness. With a strong sense of self-love and a purpose developed with our "WHY," we as women and mothers can begin to accept ourselves for who we are and what we bring to the table in every aspect of our lives. We can learn to draw healthy boundaries and put ourselves in the driver's seat of our destiny. We can stop devaluing ourselves with the game of comparison that we've played too often in the past with one another. We reclaim our power back in our society and in our homes, manifesting the same opportunity in our future generations as we teach our offspring how to develop and protect their energy. We can learn to be such a force that no external influences will stand a chance of having power over us. We can honor each other's authenticity, uniting together as women, collectively defining our important place in this world.

Overall, practicing good health and fitness is one of the greatest areas where you can demonstrate self-love. After all, "If you don't love yourself, it's impossible for you to love others. You can't give away what you don't have." (Joyce Meyer) YOU are the only one living in your shoes. YOU only have one life. YOU are one of the greatest teachers in the lives of your young children and family. If practicing self-love resulted in good health, and this good health was an insurance policy on longevity, would you invest in it? The answer comes down to YOU.

2

Why Do You Want to Be a Fit Mom?

ONE OF THE MOST POWERFUL things you can do in order to develop a great fitness plan is to develop your "WHY." Your "WHY" is the reason why your soul is calling you to make a change in the first place. It is the very thing that if you live your life without accomplishing, you may die with eternal regret... deep, I know. It's the thing we feel the most and often fear the most. It keeps us up at night when we aren't taking steps toward accomplishing it. It is that voice in our head reckoning us to make a change, the grip on our soul and the writing in the sand.

When I identified my "WHY," I was going through postpartum with my second child after a very difficult pregnancy. This second pregnancy was tough on my body. I was a few years older than my first pregnancy and was already way beyond the "peak" reproductive years at age 37. I felt sick almost the entire time, my diet consisted of foods that would settle my stomach and usually weren't the healthiest, and I didn't have the energy to make much of an effort to work out. I had been an athlete and an active, healthy person most of my life, so this stage was very hard for me to endure.

My son was delivered via a scheduled C-section; however, he ended up in the NICU after swallowing fluids and struggling to breathe shortly after being delivered. He came home weeks later after I spent days knee-deep in tears, pacing around an empty nursery, wondering when he'd be coming home. Once my son finally came home, a quiet nursery turned into a busy one with nighttime feedings, onesie changes, and many hours of no sleep. I remembered feeling a little bit of this after having my daughter, but this time around it felt more overwhelming, probably because I had two littles to care for at this time versus one. I wondered when I would have time to shower each day, get a full night's sleep, and have time to fully recover from the C-section that caused me a lot of internal pain. Then life went on; days passed... then weeks.

There's no book on how to find balance after childbirth. I remember struggling with thinking about what I needed to accomplish when I was so busy taking care of two little humans. Their needs were always a priority over mine. Thinking of myself and my needs seemed selfish. Often this was also communicated to me by other mothers who continued to put the priorities of their children above theirs, even when they may have had the time to think more about themselves.

My own mother told me that I shouldn't return to work or take on any hobby that would force my children to be without me, as I "only had one opportunity to raise them." Some of this I felt was true; however, I knew I needed a balance. I had to find myself again. I desperately wanted my body back. Deep down, I knew I needed room for self-care, yet even with knowing this, I struggled with the blurred lines of what may be deemed selfish in this pursuit. I had to take a hard look at my motives, my convictions, my values, and my innermost thoughts. I had to learn to trust myself and my instincts, as these naturally differed from what others (including my mom) thought was in the best interest for my children and me.

It was during this process that I was able to identify my "WHY" and realized that having a solid fitness life was critical for me and for my family. I realized I didn't want to emulate the same types of negative patterns I experienced in my childhood when it came to fitness. I realized that I wanted to be a healthy example to my children of what a fit mother is and should be. I wanted to live a long, healthy life so I could be there for my children and also teach them to be the same for their offspring. I knew that without accomplishing all of these things, I would live with regret. It was at that point that I decided my postpartum fitness pursuit had begun.

After identifying my "WHY," I was eager to start working toward my goals, but as life goes for a busy mom, there were setbacks. Yet, I worked hard and kept my head down. I knew it took me a long time to get out of shape and I knew it would take me as much time, if not longer, to achieve what I wanted with fitness again. Weeks turned into months, and then months turned into a year past the anniversary of establishing my "WHY." I had a consistent routine I was happy with and had achieved results, but I still wasn't completely happy with my body after having children. There were many times that I wondered if I would ever have a physique that I was happy with again as a post-partum mother, however, I had confidence in my discipline and work ethic. The one thing that I was absolutely sure of, was that I would have to take a different approach than I had in the past. I decided to challenge myself and sign up for a bodybuilding competition, to not only motivate me, but prove to myself that I could achieve this type of goal at this point in my life.

Time seemed to stand still for a while as I was busy being pregnant and having babies. I was forced to shift my focus from a different perspective and also with a different body. Something I didn't anticipate in my discovery was the number of women who didn't think that my bodybuilding goals were possible at the stage in life I was in, and also at my age. I quickly transitioned from sharing my aspirations with many to selecting the quiet few who would keep it a secret. I began to realize that I was becoming unrelatable, as society discourages women to pursue endeavors like these after the childbearing years.

This discouragement is mostly suggestive, as most fitness ads in magazines are riddled with women in their 20s with tight skin who haven't experienced the joys and pain of childbirth. And it wasn't just the ads that I was noticing at the time. I became more aware of how gyms were frequently targeting the younger crowds, how clothing stores ostracize the older crowd with styles that aren't inclusive, and how many social media platforms were only celebrating the pinnacles of fitness to a younger crowd. Although the many social media platforms I was visiting were revolutionizing the accessibility of fitness, I realized that this revolution was still targeted toward a younger one that wasn't marred with a wrinkle. All of this was incredibly discouraging. And it wasn't even the imagery that made me feel this way... it was also the lack of information that mothers, including myself, had when it came to knowing how to start their postpartum fitness journey.

During this time, I would often reminisce about my single mother and the struggles she had with maintaining her fitness after having my two sisters and me. She would spend countless hours working out and having anxiety about her diet. She talked about getting older and how it was even harder to stay fit and healthy. Sadly, she didn't have a strong support system and was left to her own devices trying to figure out how she could obtain optimal health.

Most of my childhood was filled with memories of my mother's bulimic tendencies, her discouragement around fitness, and her overall lack of self-love. Later in her life she gravitated to cosmetic procedures to temporarily fix "problem areas" and provide a sense of security. These memories were discouraging and fueled my anger about the lack of information that was out there to help mothers achieve success in fitness. My discouragement turned into anger, my anger into inspiration. I knew I had to do something to change this cycle from continuing to happen!

At the time, I felt as if society told women, "You are a mother now so nothing will ever be the same. Your fitness journey is over. There is no hope for you to achieve a fit and healthy body at this stage. Not to mention, there isn't information out there for you to make a change and you don't have the time, so you might as well give up and just be a mom. Just deal with it."

I couldn't let this be the narrative. I couldn't let this be the message to myself, to other mothers, and even to my own daughter eventually. I knew one of the biggest reasons why I faced the daily grind when I felt like I had nothing left was to ensure my kids had a solid example of fitness in their life. I didn't have this when I was young. I wanted them to know they could conquer obstacles, pick themselves up when they fell down, dig deep for that internal strength that many don't take advantage of, and create a healthy space for themselves on this planet. My example wouldn't be perfect but rather one that displayed a hard-fought journey, a constant evolution, and a positive self-discovery that would hopefully lead them to a greater sense of self-empowerment.

My past fitness experiences have allowed me to break down many dysfunctional patterns in my life and reveal a better way of doing things, creating a safe and healthy environment for myself and one that I could pass on. I knew it was one of the ultimate expressions of my human willingness to be better, to express gratitude for my abilities and shine a beacon of light in a world that is sometimes full of excuses. I wanted to be strong and I wanted my kids to be also. It was then that I truly realized at this point in my life that I knew "WHY" I wanted to be a fit mom. My "WHY" fueled my consistency with my fitness practices, and this in turn eventually resulted in me achieving my dream body composition as a mother of two and in a short period of time!

Knowing that something had to be done about the discouraging messages mothers endure when it comes to their fitness kept me up at night. My plight was to help change the negative mindset that was ingrained in the minds of many mothers after the childbearing years. I knew that if anyone needed fitness, it was the mother like I was at that time, starting a new chapter of her life and needing to understand what worked for her body at this stage of life. My soul was ignited with such vigor that I knew I couldn't rest until I became part of the solution. I knew I could be, with my previous successful fitness and athletic background. I wanted to be a part of a fitness movement that proved that mothers are capable of anything, especially in their postpartum years. It was at this point, that I began my journey that led me to not only creating this book, but also my ReShapeHER Program that became the reason why I've been able to achieve the body composition of my dreams!

Your why can be the anchor to all of your dreams if you allow it to be. By focusing on your "WHY," it allows the Universe to gravitationally pull opportunities your way. Because it is directed by your soul, its power can be so large that it can help you accomplish the seemingly impossible. This is because your "WHY" reflects what you were called to do on this Earth. It is one of your human connections with this planet. It can be your superpower if you allow it to be, as its importance takes on a charge that no opposition can destroy.

Your "WHY" will serve as the glue to your discipline when your motivation is lacking. You'll know that your goals are within reach if you're laser-focused on your "WHY." Once your "WHY" is identified, there is no denying it from that point forward. This is the point of no return. Once identified, there is an onus to do something about it and this calling can be powerful but also overwhelming. This is also the reason why many fear the process of making the effort to do this. Because of this fear, many people live their entire lives without ever knowing what their "WHY" truly is. Only those who are brave enough to identify it can and will unleash their greatest human power.

Identifying our "WHY" is not taught in school and oftentimes not even spoken about at home. Many people get caught up in pursuing things that they came across in happenstance or someone else has identified for them. They haven't taken the time to do a real soul-check to understand if these things are what truly connects them to their place in the world. In our busy world this process can be easily missed, yet it is so crucial to understanding how to achieve one's greatest dreams. There's a reason why so many people regret that they didn't have the courage to live a life that was true to themself and not the life that others expected of them. Sadly, this process happens later in life when it's near the end and they realize how many dreams may have gone unfulfilled.

Your "WHY" doesn't need to revolve around something fitness-related, but rather is the very thing that you wouldn't be able to pursue WITHOUT good health and fitness. This is the very reason why you'll be motivated to continue quality fitness practices, because without them, your "WHY" simply cannot be achieved. For example, if your "WHY" is to live a good quality of life so that you can possibly live a longer life in order to be around for your children and family, this will be the reason you'll have the ability to practice your plan on the days when you think you have nothing else to give. If this is truly your "WHY" and you're committed to it, this will be the driver for continuing your plan as long as you stay focused on it. Should you have a personal calling to pursue a big achievement in your life, knowing you cannot continue this pursuit should your health suffer, this knowledge will grip your soul and allow you to dig deep for the determination to continue practicing your fitness plan. Your "WHY" will ultimately serve as your guide to lead you to your health and fitness goals.

HOW TO IDENTIFY YOUR "WHY"

1 | Grab a Pen and Journal

One of the greatest ways we can communicate to ourselves is by writing down our thoughts. Journaling is something I've learned to do throughout my life, starting with a diary at a young age, and I've continued throughout my fitness career. By writing down our thoughts, we are able to make connections with the things we care about, would like to do, our insecurities, strengths, etc. By writing our thoughts down on paper, we are able to bring our innermost thoughts to the forefront and be able to think about them with our conscious mind.

Once they are on paper, we are then able to read them over a span of time, which includes the different perspectives we have on them each time they are revisited on paper. By writing them down, we are able to make connections to the fact that our thoughts may all connect to a main thought or surround an overall idea. As we continue to revisit our thoughts we've written on paper, we can also build on them as we generate additional thoughts that originate from the original one, oftentimes bringing us even more clarity.

2 | Ask Yourself Poignant Questions

One of the first questions you'll want to ask yourself is, "WHY do you want to be a fit mom?" You are reading this book right now because you'd like to make a change with your fitness, right? Have you asked yourself why? Why do you feel compelled to make a change? What is missing in your routine? Why does this bother you? What emotions are felt when you think of your fitness and the results that you've experienced? Questions like these will enable you to focus your thoughts on a specific subject, in this case fitness. The answers you give yourself will give you an even greater insight into the specifics on your thoughts. Write them down.

As you do this, allow yourself to be honest with your answers. If these questions strike an emotion, don't panic! This will give you an even greater clue into what your "WHY" is when it comes to fitness. If there is an uncomfortable question, ask it! Your openness and answers will drive you to where you need to be in order to uncover your "WHY." Emotional responses or those that feel like a change needs to be made are all direct paths that can lead you to your "WHY."

3 | List Your Priorities

List your greatest priorities from biggest to smallest on your paper. Starting with the biggest priorities at the top, ask yourself the following question:

"How does my fitness and/or health state positively or negatively affect this priority?"

Be honest with yourself and encourage any kind of emotion that may come along with this process. Remember, this is a deeper clue into what your "WHY" is. Remember, any type of emotional response or those that make you feel like a change needs to be made are direct paths that can lead you to your "WHY."

4 | Revisit Your Journaling

Allow yourself some time from when you journaled and completed steps #1-3. This gives you the opportunity to read your thoughts with a different perspective and also at a different time. You might be able to add to what you've written. Maybe you don't feel as strongly and realize that you may have just been emotional that day, and this thought sends you somewhere else. Maybe you realize that something about what you've written still bothers your soul and you're inclined to make a change.

Giving yourself some time to metabolize your thoughts will help you see things more clearly and with a different lens. What I like to do at this stage is write my additional thoughts down with a different-colored pen. This helps me understand if my thoughts are running parallel to my original ones or if they vary. I also allow myself to do this multiple times over, with different pen colors, to observe my thoughts on those days in the same way.

5 | Making Connections

By repeating step #4 over and over, you should then be able to make connections to the things that compel you when it comes to your fitness. Maybe you don't desire to be a Fitness influencer, but it bothers you that you don't have an overall better fitness experience and this negatively affects you and your family. Maybe you are a mother who struggles with body image post-pregnancy and you don't know how to start when it comes to fitness. Perhaps you're a mother, like I was, who struggles with the negative voice in your head that tells you that your fitness won't ever be what it once was, since going through childbirth and leading a busy life.

6 | Identify Your "WHY" and Make a Plan

By going through steps #1-5, you should be able to have a clear understanding of what your "WHY" is, but it doesn't stop there. You need to write it down so you can have it in the forefront of your mind. You need to "live it" when it comes to your fitness. Your "WHY" will be the glue to your efforts when your motivation is lacking. Your "WHY" compels you to make a change, and you know that only comes along with having a solid plan. You begin to envision your plan and you don't anticipate looking back from this point, only forward. You feel an even deeper connection to yourself and your goals by identifying your "WHY."

One of the main reasons why it's critical to develop your "WHY" when it comes to fitness is that you won't always be motivated. Some of the greatest athletes have had times that they've lacked motivation and felt like giving up. When you have days like this, your "WHY" will serve as your glue between you and your ultimate goal, helping to push you through the days that you feel like you can't make the effort. You'll realize that there isn't room for giving up, because the only thing that will result from this is zero progress toward your ultimate goal. You'll begin to familiarize yourself with the days you don't feel motivated and learn to focus on your "WHY" to pull yourself through. This is the point where you'll realize that what will really fuel your efforts with low motivation is your discipline.

HOW TO STRENGTHEN YOUR "WHY"

1 | Have a Visual Reminder

Having this visual reminder of your why not only serves as a visual reminder, but it can also help shape your thoughts and actions regarding your "WHY." When you see your "WHY" visually, it allows you to have another reminder of what you hope to achieve and what you need to work toward. I personally dedicate a small area of my closet to my fitness journey with snapshots of me along the way, including my bodybuilding medals that I can frequent often to remind myself of how far I've come and what I'm capable of.

2 | Speak Your "WHY" to Yourself and Others

This may sound crazy, but talking to yourself and pronouncing your goals by speaking them to yourself or others is very powerful. This type of practice can help us control ourselves. Talking out loud can be an extension of the silent inner talk we need to hear and can often quiet the voice of doubt. I will often perform this in the mirror and look myself in the eyes to reiterate the commitment I'm making to myself.

3 | Write Your "WHY" Down

This practice of writing down your intentions allows you to narrow your focus and provide motivation. When you develop short-term and long-term goals, this provides clarity and priority to the things that will support these goals. Through the process of nutritional tracking (as part of the ReShapeHER Program), it allows you to document your goals along with the many other methods that are available, in order to track your fitness progress. Creating a diary of your fitness journey can be very insightful as it helps you to understand your response to different approaches and what yielded you the greatest outcomes.

4 | Visualize Your "WHY"

The process of visualizing your positive fitness outcomes through your "WHY" allows you to see yourself succeeding and believing that you can—and will—achieve what you desire. I practiced the art of visualization many times through my process of developing the ReShapeHER program. I envisioned myself achieving my ideal body composition through this plan and sharing this information in this plan with others. I visualized the impact these ideas would make on others and how happy they would be to learn this information. I envisioned what this would look like on a larger scale and how mothers could be empowered with this information. I continue to visualize a fitness movement, through the education provided in this book and with the ReShapeHER program, in which we create a fit and healthier world for mothers.

The thing about fitness is that it is constantly in a fluid state. Your efforts are either making positive contributions toward your fitness or they're not. Sometimes even the smallest efforts should be celebrated, as they are still moving you in the direction of your goals. Better to be moving at 2 mph than not at all. That perspective comes down to YOU. One day won't kill your overall movement in a positive direction, but many days of bad decisions will. However, it is important to not let the bad days derail us from our overall progress. Conversely, we also can't allow a few positive days and no results bring us to the point where we give up too soon. When you have a strong vision and "WHY," you'll be able to push through the days that there is seemingly no progress being made to days that you realize you are happy you trusted the process.

We all know the phrase: "Same shit, different day!" With a strong identification of your "WHY" and a commitment to trust the process, you'll realize that this saying is just a figure of speech and not exactly true. The falsity lies in the fact that each day isn't the same because each day brings you one step closer to your ultimate goal when you're doing the work and trusting the process. Aesthetic fitness results don't happen overnight. They are not linear. They require a culmination of small, positive steps in the direction of your goal.

When it comes to motivation, we have to be sure that we aren't allowing our emotions to hinge on seeing results when we're in the process of making them. Until the point that we feel motivated, we need to learn to lean on our "WHY" to bring us to the point of motivation. Once the results are achieved and the culmination of effort is seen, it is easier to feel motivated. This is the understanding that separates those who achieve their goals in fitness and those who do not. They don't allow themselves to get discouraged in the beginning stages of pursuing their goals, but rather they keep their head down and grind for a while, raising their head when they know they've slayed these principles.

This book and my ReShapeHER program is a direct reflection of my WHY. What stirs my soul is the ability to provide fitness clarity for many mothers who struggle with knowing how to find it. This book serves as an educational outpouring of fitness truths I've learned over the years and also addresses common pitfalls that mothers have been plagued with, keeping them from reaching their fitness goals. My ReShapeHER Program provides mothers with a solid plan to combat these pitfalls and achieve the body they dream of AND DESERVE! My reason for sharing this information is to contribute to the betterment of overall health for mothers in their postpartum years. I want the next generation of women to know how to achieve optimal health and fitness. I want to cast down the negative messages that have overshadowed our society for far too long, regarding postpartum and aging bodies, their futures, and what is ultimately possible. I want my daughter to know when she becomes a mother that she can enjoy the process of that stage of her life and not fear that she won't achieve her fitness goals.

If you're reading this right now, I implore you to find your reason "WHY" you want to be a fit mom. Challenge yourself to dig deep to uncover that precious answer that stirs your soul and ignites your ability to live your fitness truth. The process may seem scary, but knowing this truth will possibly be one of your greatest areas of self-discovery. It may even allow you to love and understand yourself even better. Knowing your "WHY" can give you a laser-focus on your fitness dreams and aspirations. It will serve as your guide, your reference, and even your glue when your motivation is lacking. Trust me, finding your "WHY" could possibly be one of the greatest accomplishments you will ever make. Don't wait to find it. Once you do, read on to identify "HOW" you can reach your fitness goals with the ReShapeHER program **in as little as 4-6 weeks**!

NOTES

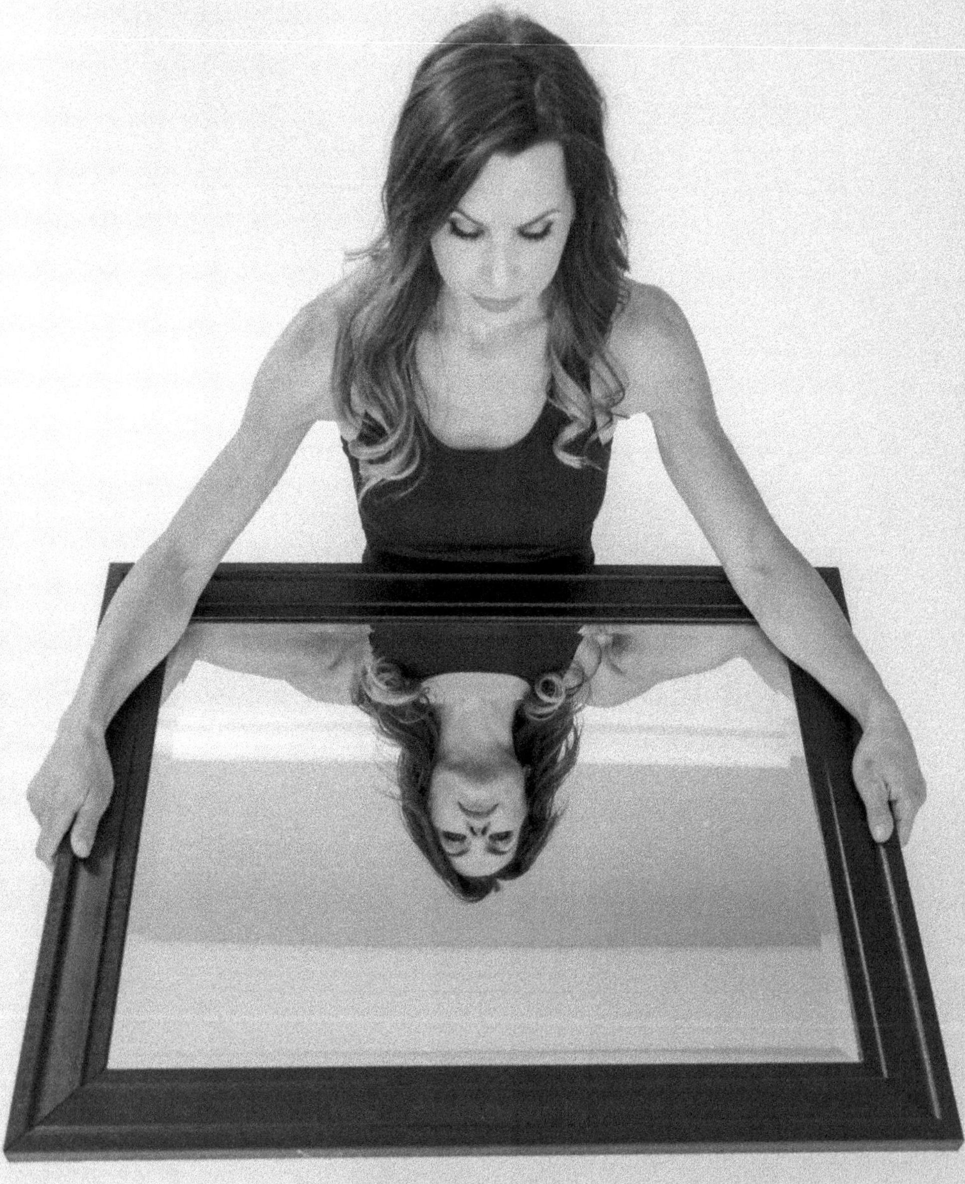

3

Mirror, Mirror on the Wall. . .

WE AS WOMEN ARE OFTEN our worst critics. It is easy to blame our society for being solely aesthetically focused when it comes to fitness, but we as women are also to blame, as we feed into our shallow association of health with our constant obsession with trying to look perfect. Since the pandemic, in which we all became even more aware of how our public images are viewed daily, this fixation on beauty and aesthetics has become even easier to adopt. Many women can even adopt dysmorphia when it comes to their body or self-image, which can drive this obsession even further.

OUR HYPER-FOCUS ON AESTHETICS

We tend to assume that if someone has a beautiful and healthy aesthetic look, then they are the definition of wellness, when in fact they may not be well at all. Although with the pressures of our changing times, in addition to the history of our gender being aesthetically revered, we as women and mothers need to take responsibility for our part in driving this aesthetic-centric trend that continues to grow.

The problem with our aesthetically focused society is that it devalues the other parts of health that make up a woman's well-being, and it is a trend that creates barriers instead of opportunities for our gender.

Our lives as women and mothers become curated to fit a mold, and this lends to gender biases, lessening our opportunities to have equal opportunities— including educational equity, which I discuss in this book. By contributing to this trend, even if unknowingly, we as women continue to pave the way for the fitness falsifications that have been the very thing to blame for our historical fitness failures. With a lack of education and a laser-focus on aesthetics alone, we aren't able to strengthen our overall wellness and place in our society.

DIMENSIONS OF WELLNESS

True wellness is the integration of both internal and external health. Both of these areas must be working in harmony to achieve the ultimate goal of being "well." There are many theories and other dimensions of wellness that experts have identified as facets of wellness that I won't discuss in detail, but the important thing to remember is that wellness isn't just defined in terms of one's physical health. As mothers, when we prioritize only our physical health and beauty alone, we overlook the other important aspects that contribute to our overall health. We also encourage others to do the same, including our offspring. We contribute to a society that is less concerned about internal health (including mental and spiritual) and instead worships beauty and ostracizes anything that is not. We become part of the societal issues we see with gender inequality by not recognizing ourselves and our wellness as a whole.

I'm sure we've all had an acquaintance who is aesthetically "fit" and beautiful, but who is completely out of balance with their other dimensions of health and extremely toxic. You see, the other aspects of wellness are sometimes hard to spot as they can't be seen or judged with the naked eye. However, they can sometimes be the greatest contributors to why someone is not healthy and isn't experiencing overall well-being. They may be aesthetically pleasing, but by the definition of wellness, they aren't "well." Yet, this woman is not given any reason to question herself or her wellness, because she is by societal standards aesthetically appealing, and through this, fitting into a false picture of health. As someone who knows her, we may label her a bitch as a result of her behavior, but on the same token, we may envy her aesthetics and credit them for this fit and healthy label she is falsely promoting. As a result, we contribute to this superficial theme, and therefore, it continues.

To be healthy, a balance of internal and external health is needed. Without a balance between these dimensions, you can't experience ultimate wellness. Your body will be too weak and you won't be able to maintain high levels of strength or energy. Without internal and external strength, you will lack productivity, having diminishing results that produce fatigue, rigidity, or failure. For example, a weak internal state will leave you overwhelmed and helpless, resulting in your body suffering the consequences. Without a sense of mental well-being, feelings can be suppressed or avoided, leading to possible disease and dysfunction. Spiritual imbalances with our internal health can often result in disconnections between your inner being and those around you.

It is important that in a successful fitness plan there is time dedicated to all aspects of wellness, not just the physical component. Each part should be deemed separate but inclusive when it comes to understanding their overall contributions to someone's overall wellness. Consistent practice toward strengthening both parts should be done to ensure that someone achieves balance. This balance will be the key to ensuring that they are making the greatest achievement when it comes to their overall fitness goals.

Good overall health requires the practice of good habits. These habits, when done consistently over time, are what lead to positive results. Things such as healthy eating, getting quality sleep, drinking plenty of water, exercising, etc., are all ways we can make notable changes to our physical health in a positive way. Physical health, although it takes time, can be seen with the naked eye, which is satisfying in regards to quantifying results in terms of effort over time. With consistent practice, we can make visual changes to our bodily tone and the condition of our skin. Additionally, we can also quantify results we make in terms of endurance, strength, flexibility, and cardiovascular health through our physical efforts of reaching goals, hitting benchmarks, etc., with our fitness training.

As mothers, the external part of our physical health dimension can often be the part that we are consumed with the most. As our bodies endure changes that are needed in order to grow and labor a healthy child, our aesthetics can change and often bring frustration to us as these changes can seem very unpleasant and foreign (especially when experienced for the first time). This is why during pregnancy and during the postpartum phase, it is critical to remember that our external part of our physical health is only one dimension of health (one that requires these temporary changes to occur). We need to understand that it behooves us to often shift our focus to strengthening our internal health to ensure a successful pregnancy and postpartum phase. This isn't to say that we shouldn't consider the external part of our physical health dimension, but rather not allow it to derail us from making progress with the other dimensions of health.

As women and mothers, we need to have the confidence in knowing that we will endure changes with the external part of our physical health that are out of our control, but understand that this is part of the process and that we will eventually reclaim the control we once had, after we let our bodies do what they need to do in order to be successful. Of course, this is easier said than done, but as mothers, we need to work toward this type of thinking. What ultimately calms the fear and brings us to the point of thinking in this way is through education—knowing what to do in order to reclaim control of the external part of our physical health when the time comes to do so. This education surrounding how women can do this is so desperately needed and serves as one of my greatest motivations for writing this book.

IMPORTANCE OF MENTAL HEALTH

Mental health is an important part of our internal health. It can often be the most complicated aspect of health in that its overall contribution can't be easily seen or evaluated. It affects how we act, think, and feel. It determines how we handle social situations and interact with others, our behaviors, and how we handle life's stresses. Taking successful steps to ensure a mental health balance not only includes the practice of communication and relationships with others (including oneself), but also aspects of physical health practice. Practicing a balance with mental health requires practices that also balance physical health such as exercise, sleep, proper diet, leisurely activities, and relaxation/rest. Conversely, physical health also requires practices that balance mental health such as communication with others (including oneself).

The development of mental strength is so important, as our minds give us that inner quality to be able to push past obstacles and achieve our greatest dreams. Our minds allow us to respond positively and successfully to adversity and failure. Ultimately, our minds can be our capitation point to our potential, whether great or small. Having a positive headspace is absolutely critical when trying to work toward fitness goals and avoiding derailment. Your mind is arguably the body's most powerful organ. It is the epicenter for all of the things that control and coordinate our actions, our feelings, and our thoughts, and it enables us to have memories.

If you think about it, the brain is the one organ that allows us to be all of the things that make us human. The mind can ultimately create a thought and turn it into reality. Knowing how powerful the mind can be in this regard, it is essential that we don't allow negative thoughts to take over our headspace. Negativity, in and of itself, is viral. It can be insidious and replicate rapidly, with one negative thought easily turning into hundreds in a short period of time. It can infect and invade even positive thoughts and ultimately take over our entire viewpoint of the world if we let it. It may not even reflect the reality of our circumstances, but due to its infectious nature it can quickly become it. It can also infect others and cause the same to happen to them. Negative thoughts are also very limiting and non-productive, which is why it's so antagonistic to our fitness as mothers.

Sometimes as mothers, we ourselves struggle with our inner child in finding the mental strength to overcome adversity, even the kind we may pose upon ourselves. We are often so critical of ourselves that we allow our internal criticisms to derail us of our potential successes. We allow the voice inside our head to become loud and negative, limiting our potential and keeping us shackled to unproductive ideas (such as the idea that as mothers, we don't have the ability to achieve fitness success after pregnancy). It is critical that we continue to work on strengthening our mental health so that we can achieve our dreams and be able to teach our children to do the same!

One way a mother can work to strengthen her mental health is by developing a successful routine. It is important to develop one, as this practice provides structure to your day. It serves as a reminder of what your priorities are and the importance of accomplishing what's on your to-do list in order to complete them. A routine can drive happiness in that it can give you a feeling of satisfaction that you have aligned your daily plans to your goals and a sense of accomplishment once you've achieved them. It also drives consistency, as a routine is something that is practiced often and becomes part of one's lifestyle. Once established, it allows you the opportunity to possibly ward off life's distractions as the practice of your routine becomes ingrained. Additionally, after practicing a successful routine and seeing health results from it, this may also drive motivation to continue it, adding to the consistency in its practice.

THE FLUIDITY OF HEALTH

Regardless of the health dimension being discussed, it is also important to remember that each dimension is continually in a fluid state. Health, whether external or internal, should never be taken advantage of as it can be quickly lost (I think we can all appreciate this after experiencing the pandemic). Because of the fluidity of health, it is also something that can be changed from bad to good; however, it depends on the circumstance and it also takes time. Because of this state of flux, good health is temporary in nature and has to be exercised. This is part of what makes health a journey, not a race that, once ended, we take our medals home and forever call ourselves by a title. Good health can be the most fulfilling experience, yet bad health can be your worst nightmare. Some of the greatest lessons we learn in our journey of health can also include some of our biggest failures. How we pick ourselves back up and carry on after these failures is what defines who we are and what results we experience afterward.

As mothers, we can't continue to allow our society to try and convince us that exercising just one dimension of health (the physical dimension with a large emphasis on aesthetics alone) is what ultimately makes us fit and healthy. We need to remember that our wellness consists of so much more than that! We have to remember that when we are working to achieve our desired aesthetics, we need to place just as much emphasis on the other dimensions of health, because in total they define our overall wellness. All three dimensions work in synergy, making us the strong and amazing mothers that we are. After all, it takes a shitload of strength to bring life into this world, and we have all done it! So let's give ourselves a high-five and move forward knowing that we have the ability to work on our strength in many ways, outside of just what we see in the mirror.

The REFRAME

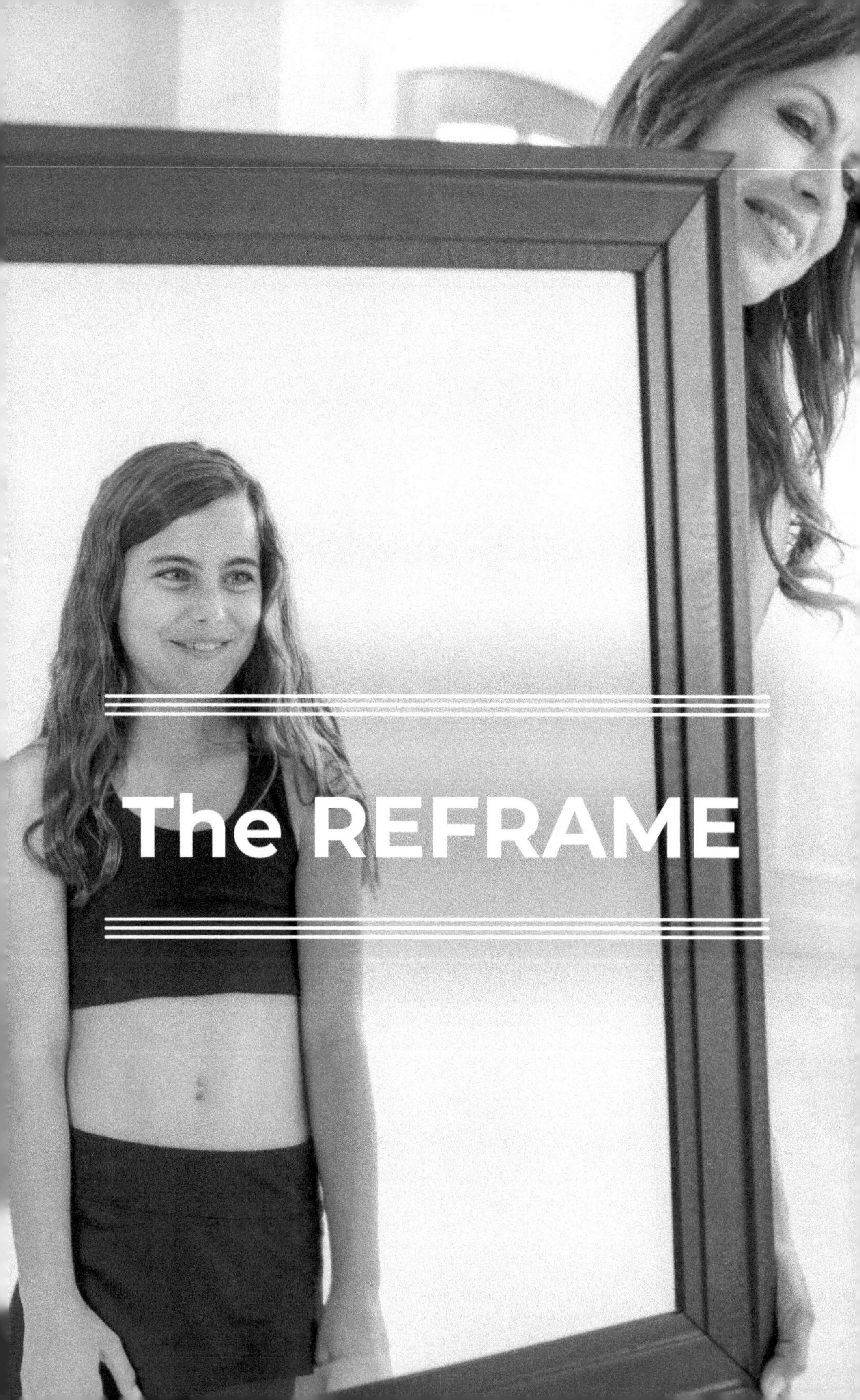

4

Simplifying the Science of Nutrition and Weight Loss

WE'VE ALL HEARD THE SAYING "You are what you eat!" This old saying couldn't be more true! I'll spend this chapter explaining just this, but first, I must talk about the simple calorie and how it's also defined in terms of a macro.

You may be wondering what the heck I'm talking about at this point. I completely understand. Our current education surrounding health and fitness doesn't discuss these types of things. Sure, we may have learned about the basic food groups, but are we truly understanding how these groups are broken down into fats, proteins, and carbs and what they mean in terms of supporting a healthy body? Nope. Unless you are a fitness competitor, nutritionist, or health coach, or you are lucky enough to have an occupation that encourages you to understand health and fitness, or you just have an interest in understanding these things, you may not have ever had this type of education. This is one of the main reasons why I wrote this book: to help women (especially mothers) like yourself understand the science behind nutrition and fitness so they can achieve their fitness goals.

In order to reach our goals as mothers, it is critical to understand the basic principles that will support our understanding of nutrition and fitness. In the following chapters, I will save you both **TIME** and **MONEY** as I simplify many of these principles for you. In order for us to know how and why we apply these principles to our individual goals, it is critical to take the time to educate ourselves on them. Once you have the baseline knowledge of nutrition and fitness that is found in this chapter, you'll be able to start applying this information to your personal goals with the ReShapeHER program and get results in as little as 12 weeks!

THE SIMPLE CALORIE

The calorie (also used interchangeably with the word kcal) is defined in the Oxford dictionary as "a unit of energy; the amount of heat needed to raise the temperature of a quantity of water by one degree." The first time I heard of the term calorie, I was in high school chemistry class. I expanded my knowledge of a calorie later in college, but only from a biological standpoint and not one that I was able to apply to health and fitness. Sure I learned to read labels and understand that the more calories a food was, the longer it would take to burn, but I wasn't able to expand on this knowledge and use it to apply to advance my fitness. Matter of fact, when I was in college (and I am probably dating myself), learning to read labels had just become a new "thing."

Prior to attending in 1995, nutritional information was not always required on packaged foods and beverages. The U.S. Nutrition Facts label first appeared in 1994 and was actually revised in 2016 (there is now an even newer, updated version that was required on products as of January 1, 2020). I was only an early adopter to label reading, with my experience as a collegiate athlete and as an undergraduate of biology. Both of these things, and my interest in general health information, kept me interested in surfing this new tide of information that was developing in the world of health.

I remember going shopping at the grocery store in college, avoiding any item that had a higher caloric content listed on its package, assuming they were the "bad" foods since it would take me more energy to burn off. What I failed to realize was the quality of the high-calorie content, as well as the lack of quality of the lower-calorie foods I was ingesting. The items that I was snacking on were completely void of essential nutrients and vitamins my body so desperately needed to be a successful and healthy athlete. Sadly, I didn't understand this nor was this education being taught. I was mainly motivated by the pressure to stay lean as an athlete as well as fulfilling the social pressures of being a young woman.

What I didn't understand during this time was that the amount of each macronutrient, and how each one is weighted in terms of your diet, is critical in having a successful diet. Whether your goal is to maintain, lose, or gain weight, understanding these values will enable you to tailor a nutritional program that is the best one for YOU. This is the one principle area that can allow anyone to have total control of their diet and their goals. However, it takes time to understand how much of each macro an individual needs and in what amount. Additionally, these values also change over time depending on your body composition and goals. I will go into each macro and its value in a later chapter in this book.

Knowing the value of each macronutrient and how much you need in your diet is critical, but it is also important to understand the principle of overall "Energy Balance" and how these macros will ultimately be consumed or stored by your body. When speaking of this principle, it is true that every calorie matters. What's left at the end of the day after consumption is what either drives the storage of calories and/or also drives the deficit of calories that have been created. There is not a calorie that doesn't matter, in that the body is doing one of two things with them—storing them (which results in fat gain unless they are expended) or dealing with a deficit (resulting in fat loss over time).

TDEE (Total Daily Energy Expenditure)

Your total daily energy expenditure (TDEE) over the course of a day is actually composed of four different values that make up its 100%. I like to think of my daily calories, or TDEE, like I would a daily paycheck. Calories that are under-consumed (or in this analogy, money not spent), allow you to save them for another day or put towards a calorie deficit (resulting in weight loss). Calories that are over-consumed (or in this analogy, money over spent), require you to borrow from another day or contribute towards a calorie surplus (resulting in weight gain). Calories that are consumed at or around one's TDEE on a daily basis, allow someone to maintain their current weight, as this doesn't contribute towards a calorie deficit or surplus.

Creating a calorie deficit, maintaining one's calories at their TDEE (daily calorie limit), or creating a surplus, are all done by manipulating two things: nutrition and movement. You can create a deficit or surplus through one of these alone or you can manipulate both to reach your fitness goals. When it comes to creating a deficit, some would argue that it's easier to accomplish this through nutrition versus exercise, as it's easier to consume less food or drinks versus trying to achieve the amount of movement that is required to equal the same amount of calories you are trying to expend. Others would say that it's easier done with exercise, as they might feel it's harder to eat a lesser amount of calories to achieve their goal. The remainder of people may feel like with nutrition and exercise collectively, they can successfully achieve a calorie deficit. Conversely, when it comes to creating a surplus, most would consider consuming more calories as an avenue to successfully completing this goal. However, a surplus can also be supported by lessening one's movement throughout the day, to support a lesser number of calories being expended. How someone achieves a calorie deficit or surplus is highly individualized. Also, the only way to understand how accurately we do this, is by tracking our nutrition and exercise (a practice the ReShapeHER program supports and is discussed in much greater detail later in this book).

The activities that allow us to expend our calories consumed through our food and drinks, are grouped into four categories: REE, NEAT, TEF and EAT. REE (otherwise known as your resting energy expenditure) calories are those that you burn just being alive and functioning. These REE calories make up 70% of your overall calorie expenditure each day. Things such as breathing, sweating, sleeping, etc. are all under this type of expenditure.

Second to your REE is your NEAT (non-exercise activity), which makes up 15% of your daily expenditure. Things such as walking, doing household chores, taking stairs versus the elevator, standing versus sitting, and just being "active" all count toward your NEAT expenditure (I discuss this key area in more depth in a later chapter). Your NEAT expenditure is accomplished through your daily movements and is categorized as unplanned exercise.

Your TEF (your thermic effect of food) calories are those your body uses to metabolize your food. This makes up 10% of your overall expenditure and is similar to your REE, in that your body automatically does this on its own. Additionally, your REE and TEF make up your BMR (your basal metabolic rate; the minimum number of calories that your body needs to function at rest). Calorie calculators are based on your calculated BMR (basal metabolic rate) value. This value is then multiplied by your activity level (ranging from sedentary to extremely active), to determine your overall calorie consumption per day.

It is important to note that your EAT (exercise activity thermogenesis or "planned exercise") makes up only 5% of your TDEE as compared to the other three categories. This is your planned workout for the day, including both cardiovascular and resistance training activities. Due to its lesser contribution as compared to the other three categories, you can see how it can be easy to assume that our planned exercise for the day may or may not be contributing as much as we'd originally thought towards our overall daily calories. However, our planned exercise is critical, in that we wouldn't obtain the benefits from our Resistance training and additional cardiovascular activities without it.

TDEE

The chart below depicts the four categories that contribute to our TDEE:

REE*	70%
NEAT	15%
TEF*	10%
EAT	5%
TDEE	100%

**TEF and REE both contribute to one's BMR (Basal Metabolic Rate). The BMR value refers to the amount of energy the body needs to maintain homeostasis.*

When it comes to our overall daily movements (both EAT and NEAT) your EAT activities can count towards your NEAT activities and vise-versa. However, there is a caveat. If you complete a great fitness session for the day, (satisfying your EAT goal), but sit on the couch the rest of the day, you wouldn't be contributing towards your NEAT calorie-expenditure (which as a reminder, is a whopping 15%). Conversely, if you had an active day and accomplished a large NEAT value, you might have had a large contribution towards your overall daily calorie expenditure but weren't able to take advantage of the additional health benefits that would have resulted from completing a planned EAT session. This is the reason why BOTH types of activities (both EAT and NEAT) are important to have as a part of a successful fitness plan.

So, you can see that even without considering macronutrients and their values at this point, you can see the areas that are the greatest contributors to your energy expenditure per day and what areas you can make an impact on (NEAT and EAT). Knowing that calories are either stored or burned, if your goal is weight loss, you will want to create a calorie "deficit" (consume fewer calories per day) in either of these two areas when it comes to your exercise. If your goal is maintenance, you'll want to keep your calories steady. Lastly, if you want to gain lean muscle tissue, you'll want to create a surplus (consume additional calories).

DIETING

Creating a calorie deficit is not only done by impacting your NEAT and EAT activity and movement levels, but it is also done with diet. Consuming fewer calories will enable the body to have less of an ability to store, therefore creating an environment for fat loss. However, when doing this, it is important to understand that there are suboptimal levels by which calories can be too low, therefore creating an environment for not only fat loss but also muscle loss. This is why it's important when trying to lose fat and develop or maintain muscle that a conservative deficit is created in order to prevent this muscle loss from happening. Muscle takes a lot of time and effort to put on, which is why any loss can be very disappointing.

Spot Reduction

The idea of reducing body fat in a particular area with dieting, is simply not possible. We can't control where our bodies lose fat. All we can control is our body composition, in terms of how we can reduce our overall body fat mass through our fitness efforts, along with balancing this with our lean muscle tissue. Our physical activities and overall movements, can help burn body fat and preserve muscle mass, which helps us achieve better body compositions. Additionally, our diets are also key, in making sure we aren't contributing to an environment that derails these efforts with an overconsumption of calories, not enough calories or the wrong type of calories.

"Get In, Get Out" Goal with Dieting

The overall takeaway with dieting, or putting oneself in a calorie deficit, is to always remember that it's not intended to be a forever practice and there are downfalls in making it one, (that I'll discuss later in this book).

A healthy weight and realistic fitness plan should be the goal, and a diet (or calorie restriction) should only be practiced until that goal is achieved. The "Get In, Get out" motto is one that the ReShapeHER program supports, to encourage a mother to think of a dieting phase as temporary, and one that she should enter, although conservatively, but adhere to successful practices so she can exit as soon as she's able. A mother's long-term goal should be one in which she is supporting her current body composition.

Unfortunately, our society and social media make it seem as though a diet is an acceptable practice all the time. The term "diet" is used so much in our society (especially with women) that it's easy to think you need to be on one when your goal should be focused on muscle development and not fat loss. It is really important to know that a successful fitness plan is fluid, changing as your body does, allowing you to achieve the best version of YOU.

Metabolic Adaptation

The body is really good at adapting to a changing environment, which is also another reason why it's good to have "seasons" in a fitness plan, (which I'll discuss later in much greater detail). When you drive your calories down, your body quickly learns how to function on fewer calories, also driving your metabolism down in the process. Another thing that many women don't take into consideration is that in addition to this adaptation, a lower weight will also require fewer calories to function (less weight equals a lower BMR). This lower-calorie ceiling will need to be maintained in order to maintain the lower body weight that was achieved. If you couple this with the body's ability to adapt at a lower calorie rate, you can see how dieting for a long period of time can ultimately drive calories really low. At this point, many women may blame hormones or aging as the reason for feeling like they gain weight when they eat less than what they did before; however, what they don't take into consideration are the dietary practices they've been doing that led them to this point.

Metabolic adaptation is the reason why diets may work initially, but over time they start to become unsuccessful. I know many women who complain that strict dieting or skipping meals has worked at one point in their earlier life, only to have it be unsuccessful later in their life or actually backfire. This is due in large part to metabolic adaptation, if they've constantly been in and out of dieting phases without successfully leaving them and spending time correcting the adaptation that has taken place. Oftentimes, the more aggressive the diet approach, the quicker the adaptation. Without correcting this adaptation, the body learns to function on fewer calories consumed. As a result, this may possibly steal calories from your lean muscle tissue in the process, leaving you with less of it and a body composition that lacks more tone than the one you had before. Not only does constant dieting cause this metabolic adaptation and muscle loss to occur, but it also wreaks havoc on your body in terms of stress, adrenal fatigue, nutritional deficits, and many other things that can derail you from reaching your fitness goals.

Metabolic adaptation is also to blame and the reason why weight loss can seem so difficult at times, lending itself to not being a linear process. For example, this is why a woman might find it easier to lose an initial 10 pounds of body weight (with a goal of losing 20 overall) yet struggle to lose the last 10. This weight will eventually come off with a great plan and being practiced with consistency, but she may experience weight plateaus and spikes along the way, before reaching her ultimate goal.

The more the body is challenged from being in the area of "status quo" it once was in, the more it will respond through metabolic adaptation in order to bring itself back to that point (even if you may have been heavier or leaner prior to starting a calorie deficit). Depending on your dieting history, you may or may not have to work even harder than before to lose body weight and do it within the same period of time. I know from personal experience that my efforts in trying to lose the same 10 pounds, even beginning with the same body weight, has taken me anywhere from five weeks to three months. The key to having success with weight loss is to understand that it isn't linear. It is a process that requires a great fitness plan along with patience and consistency, until your fitness goals are met.

It is important to keep in mind that when we diet down too aggressively and consume fewer calories over time, we will often feel less energetic and, therefore, contribute less to our movements for the day. These values contribute to 20% of their overall calorie expenditure, so if they are lower than what they were before, fewer calories will be required as fewer are being burned. This is also another area that hormones and aging are sometimes to blame, when in fact, it is our lack of movement (as a result of our lowered energy levels) that is often to blame.

Metabolic adaptation is the reason why when dieting down, you don't want to do it too aggressively, and for too long, in order to keep your calorie ceiling as high as possible yet achieving healthy and effective results. This is the reason why the ReShapeHER program supports a conservative approach to dieting, as well as a quick exit once a mother's goals are achieved. The ReshapeHER program focuses a mother on supporting her weight loss efforts with tailored, nutrient values that encourage wholesome eating, allowing her to feel healthy and satiated. When a mother is focused on eating the right foods, in the right amounts, this will allow her to reach her fitness goals when it comes to nutrition. By practicing the nutritional part of the ReShapeHER program, a woman can confidently know that she is contributing to her nutritional and weight loss goals, if she practices it consistently.

BODY WEIGHT VS. BODY FAT

When making efforts to achieve weight loss and combating metabolic adaptation, it is also imperative that a woman understands the difference between body weight and percentage body fat. This is the area the scales don't delineate and can often muddy the waters if our goals are only incorporating hitting a "target" number on the scale versus looking at our body composition as a whole. For example, I have been the same "scale" weight with a percentage body fat of both 22% and 10%. The reason for this is because I simply had more muscle making up my scale weight at 10% versus 22%. My body composition with my percentage body fat at 10% was more aesthetically appealing, as I had great "tone" with more muscle development being seen underneath my body fat. This is how the average scale can be very misleading and why fitness goals shouldn't be based on body weight and need to include the analysis of one's body composition (I discuss this further in future chapters).

Many of us women allow our scale weight to dictate our progress. This is a dangerous practice. Scale weight can vary quite a bit throughout the week (which is why I always recommend to clients taking a weekly average and plotting it, to understand your weekly average). Weight loss, in general, is not a linear process. This is the reason why it's critical to exercise patience as multiple weigh-ins should be evaluated each week, to truly understand what weight a mother truly is. Things like inflammation, our hormones fluctuations, our sodium intake, our macronutrients ingested, our resistance-training efforts, going to a sauna, or even having a bowel movement can impact our scale weight. This is the reason why the ReShapeHER program incorporates other types of measurements into the plan, such as a body composition analysis, which can be a much better indicator of progress versus the average scale.

Understanding Body Composition

It is essential for a successful fitness plan to include analyzing a woman's body composition as the primary tool used to determine her progress in lieu of the common scale. The reason for this is because it considers all of the variables that make up weight: muscle mass, body fat mass, bone, and water (all four contribute to a woman's overall scale weight). Without these values, a woman is not able to understand where she's making progress when it comes to increasing or decreasing her muscle mass or body fat, which inadvertently contributes to her overall body composition (and can determine her state of "tone").

Relying on scale weight alone is one-dimensional and simply can't be used as a predictor of fitness progress. However, it can be used as a tool to determine possible trends when it comes to the gain or loss of overall body weight, as this overall value is indicative of body composition changes.

BMI (Body Mass Index)

Another area that can often not be a good predictor of health is BMI (body mass index). Although this index is used in the medical community to screen weight categories that may lead to health problems, it doesn't diagnose the true body fat for an individual. This is because it only takes into consideration a person's weight (in kilograms or pounds). That number is divided by the square root of their height (in meters or feet). This is the reason why a female bodybuilder can actually have a higher BMI than a woman who doesn't have as healthy of a body composition. The bodybuilder simply weighs more for her height because of her muscle mass, yet has a healthier body composition compared to another female because her muscle mass to body fat ratio is better.

MACRONUTRIENTS

Calories do matter and reign supreme in terms of overall energy goals for a fitness plan; however, the macronutrients that make up these calories (which I will discuss in future chapters) need to be considered in order to reach our fitness goals. Additionally, it is critical to understand the energy balance these macronutrients contribute to our overall daily intake of calories. Understanding these macronutrients and the energy they provide is how you can get the most out of your fitness plan in terms of providing your body the fuel it needs to survive, function, stay active, grow, and also lose unnecessary fat.

There are seven major classes of nutrients: proteins, fats, carbohydrates, dietary fiber, minerals, vitamins, and water. All food is composed of mainly three different types of macronutrients: proteins, fats, and carbohydrates. They are all critical in our diets for different reasons and are required for our human bodies to orchestrate a range of physiological functions each day. Understanding these macronutrients and the role they serve in any diet is the key to knowing what types of foods, and how much, to consume for one's fitness success. Considering how important these nutrients are to our diet, you would think more teaching surrounding these nutrients and overall nutrition would be a greater focus in our educational system.

Nutritional education in this nation varies among schools, and the time allotted to talking about healthy eating in an already packed school day is a big hurdle. Personally, I don't recall having any formal education on nutrition until I entered college for my bachelor's degree (and a large part I'll credit to being a biology major). Other than the Basic Food Group (which my parents would often reference growing up), I never remember having a conversation around food values and macronutrients. The only memories I have about nutrition from my childhood were the fears of shunning certain foods that were labeled as "bad," as they were depicted as having too much sugar or fat or posed a threat in raising my cholesterol (even the wholesome egg was avoided).

I learned to avoid these foods but never had a deeper understanding of the threats (or non-threats) they posed to my diet and overall health. I learned to avoid these foods when, in fact, many of them were chock full of important macronutrients that could have been beneficial to my diet as a growing adolescent and young adult. Oftentimes, I wonder if my autoimmune disease could have been avoided had I received an education about nutrition at a younger age (through the educational system or my parents), and applied this education to my diet at that time.

According to the CDC, the number of children and adolescents who are considered obese has more than tripled since the 1970s.[1,2] Data from 2015–2016 found almost one in five Americans between six and 19 were obese. Most children don't meet the recommended intake of fruits and vegetables. Sugary beverages reportedly account for 10%

of U.S. children's caloric intake. Empty calories from sugars and fats account for about 40% of American kids' daily calories on average.[3] Today, nutritional education is more relevant than ever.

Most of what I learned about nutrition was from college, but admittedly, the plethora of information I know today has come from my own personal experience, studies, and fitness relationships. I realized with my recent experience competing in the bodybuilding world, that there's a large gap between the overall fitness understanding of fitness professionals versus the layperson. Most of the common knowledge that we have been taught, or currently exists, doesn't apply in terms of getting amazing fitness results.

Many recommendations provided in our current fitness education have become archaic in the common world and desperately need updating. For example, general requirements for macronutrients for an adult female would need to be adjusted if the goal was to maximize muscle growth, achieve fat loss, and result in overall body "tone." Additionally, some aspects of the fitness industry have provided confusion in our modern-day society, with the popularity of fad diets and false promises on how women can achieve an ideal body composition with these things. The internet is also infiltrated with pictures of so-called healthy women in peak condition, making it seem as though this is achievable with the basic information that is out there for the common person. We are currently in a world of fitness illusion, which is sad considering fitness education should be something that is attainable for every person. Considering all of this, you can see why we have an obesity epidemic on our hands and generations of mothers who are confused about how they can achieve optimal fitness.

All of the above, and more, was the reason why I looked forward to writing this chapter. In my experience, I've learned that we've done a good job complicating the world of fitness and a lot of success can come from just going back to the basics. I've also learned that there are many influencers out there who wouldn't like you to know this, because ignorance allows you to be reliant on them and the services they offer. After all, in the world of training and coaching, client continuum is everything. The honest motivation for any good coach should be the desire to instill principles in the minds of those they work with so they don't need them at a later point. Their goals should be to empower the people they work with so they can take control of their own fitness goals. Be careful as this is not the motivation for every coach and trainer!

When first doing research on macros, I remember asking myself if the overall daily caloric intake (TDEE) my body required mattered more than my required macros percentages I was supposed to consume. The answer is this: overall calories reign supreme. However, the amount of each macronutrient that comprises this overall calorie intake is key, in that these amounts will ultimately determine how, when, and if you reach your goal. For example, one of the most important macros is protein. Without ingesting enough protein, you won't be able to develop muscle tissue that will greatly add to your overall body composition. Another example is without fats, your hormones can't function at their greatest capacity without enough of them ingested. Your overall caloric intake will ultimately determine how many calories you can spend on all three; all of which are important to understand when it comes to your fitness goals.

Protein

Before I dive into how to calculate how much of each macronutrient a mother would need based on her TDEE, I'll quickly review each macro. As I stated above, proteins are essential to building muscle mass. They are commonly found in animal products, which is why it's harder for vegetarians to reach their required amounts. However, they are also present in many non-animal sources, such as nuts and legumes. The RDA recommendation for protein is 0.8g/kg of protein per day for both males and females, with a recommended acceptable macronutrient range (AMDR) of 10–35% a day.[4] There are caveats to this requirement. Some researchers have suggested that older females may have higher needs for protein consumption at around 1.2g/kg, as the elderly should ingest more to prevent muscle loss and osteoporosis.

An article posted by the National Institute of Health suggests that higher considerations of protein may support muscle mass maintenance and also bone health when calcium and vitamin D intakes are adequate.[5] I know from my own personal experience in the bodybuilding world that upwards of 2g/kg per day or more, may be suggested for women to maximize the process of muscle growth.

Regardless of need requirements, it's important to note how critical protein is in one's diet. The body contains thousands of different proteins, each with unique functions. The building blocks to proteins are nitrogen-containing molecules called amino acids. Body cells have all 20 amino acids available in ample amounts, and you can make an infinite number of proteins. Nine of these 20 amino acids are essential, meaning you must get them from your diet. Some proteins are enzymes, hormones, antibodies. Some provide structure (such as collagen). Some maintain fluid balance; they can transport nutrients and other compounds in and out of the cell. They can maintain the body's acid-base balance and they serve as a backup source of energy. They provide the body with 4 cal/g of energy; however, providing the body energy like carbohydrates is not their primary role. Each gram of protein ingested provides the body with four calories per gram.

Carbohydrates

Carbohydrates are another unique macronutrient. The basic structure of a carbohydrate is a sugar molecule, so they are classified based on how many sugar molecules they contain. Simple carbohydrates are referred to as sugars. They are naturally present in fruit, milk, and other unprocessed foods. Plant carbohydrates can be refined into table sugar and syrup, which can then be added to foods such as sodas, desserts, and more. Simple carbohydrates may be single sugar molecules (called monosaccharides) or two monosaccharides joined together (called disaccharides). Glucose, a monosaccharide, is the most abundant sugar molecule and is the preferred energy source for the brain.

Two common disaccharides in food are sucrose (common table sugar) and lactose (found in milk). Complex carbohydrates are ones that contain more than two sugar molecules; short chains being called oligosaccharides and chains of more than ten monosaccharides linked together being called polysaccharides (which may be hundreds and even thousands of glucose molecules long). The way in which these glucose molecules are linked together makes them either digestible (starch) or non-digestible (fiber). The important thing to note is that glycogen is the storage form of glucose in humans and other animals. It's not a dietary source of carbohydrates because it's quickly broken down. Glycogen is important to understand in terms of where it is stored (muscle tissue and liver) and its role in the body.

Ultimately, carbohydrates serve as fuel for your body and are the preferred energy source for the brain, nervous system, and red blood cells. Carbs also spare protein in the body. Without glycogen being stored in the tissues, your body will grab from your protein stores in your diet (if available) or from your muscles and organs, converting it into glucose. Additionally, carbohydrates prevent ketosis. Ketosis can cause the blood to become too acidic and the body to become dehydrated when too little carbohydrate is consumed. The cells need carbohydrates to break down fats; otherwise, they can build to unsafe levels within the body as the liver will produce ketone bodies.

The RDA for carbohydrates for children and adults is 130g, with a recommended acceptable macronutrient distribution range (AMDR) of 45–65% a day.[6] Most Americans fall within this range at 50%; however, the type of carbohydrates chosen may not be the healthiest. The WHO recently updated its guidelines in 2023, giving specific suggestions for the first time, as it relates to vegetables, fruits, and fiber for children and adolescents. It suggests at least 400g of vegetables and fruits per day for ages 10 and older, as well as 25g a day of naturally occurring dietary fiber.[7] All of these carbohydrate types provide 4 calories per gram, which is similar to protein (also 4 calories per gram).

Carbohydrates that are labeled "healthy" are considered this by their nutrient density. The best evaluation of carbohydrate-rich foods that can be used is the Glycemic Index. This index score indicates the increase in blood glucose from a single food containing 50 grams of carbohydrate compared to 50 grams of pure glucose (which has a GI score of 100). Foods that are slowly digested and absorbed have a low GI score using this index; faster-digested foods have a higher GI score. It is suggested that diets based on lower GI scores may be linked to lower risks of diabetes, obesity, and heart disease; however, other studies fail to show this link. Some may say that this GI score oversimplifies good nutrition. However, one can't argue that a handful of fresh cherries picked off the tree has better nutrition than a package of processed crackers (even though the cherries may provide the body a higher amount of glucose). This is why regardless of its GI score, it's important to focus on the nutrient density of foods.

Carbohydrates, over the years, have received a bad name for the very thing that they provide: glucose. I myself have gone on low-carb diets, demonizing their ingestion at times, only to find that by shunning this important macronutrient, I suffered brain fog and was void of important nutrients of benefit to a healthy diet. One of these nutrients needed in a healthy diet is fiber. Without it, we wouldn't have enough phytonutrients, the compounds found in plant foods (such as lycopene, lutein, and indole-3-carbinol) that are linked to stimulating the immune system and preventing damage to the DNA. Additionally, fiber-rich foods are linked to lower risks of coronary heart disease, stroke, hypertension, diabetes, and obesity.[8] The NIH suggests that consumption of whole grains, dietary fiber, and dairy products is protective, which is the direct opposite of what a diet of red meat, processed foods, and fat-rich diets provide.[9]

When it comes to resistance training and bodybuilding in general, carbohydrates are revered as the "energy providers." It is essential for women to have an ample amount of carbohydrates to keep up with their energy demands. It is absolutely possible for a woman to understand how to choose healthy, nutrient-dense carbohydrates in order to do this and not gain unnecessary fat. Through proper education, women can learn how to obtain great tone by knowing how to utilize fibrous carbohydrates to provide food volume, using this to their advantage while they continue to benefit from all of the essential nutrients that carbohydrates provide. Some women may prefer a slightly lower-carb diet than others, and prefer trading their calorie intake of carbohydrates to that of fat. Fat is also an energy source; however, it is more calorie-dense than carbohydrates (9kcal/g versus 4kcal/g), so understanding this difference is critical in meeting fitness goals when doing this.

Fats

Fats are the third macronutrient I'll discuss in this chapter. Fats and oils (collectively known as lipids) contain fatty acids. The World Health Organization (WHO) reaffirmed in its updated guidelines for 2023 that no more than 30% of daily adult diets should consist of fats.[10] The acceptable macronutrient distribution range (AMDR) is 20–35% for women ages 19 years and older, and 30–40% for children (depending on age). Each gram of fat provides the body with nine calories of energy, which is over two times that of a gram of protein or carbohydrate.

Fats are categorized by their types: saturated, trans, and unsaturated. Saturated fats are not needed in the diet as your body can make all of the ones that it needs. According to the Dietary Guidelines for Americans 2010, we should limit our intake of saturated fatty acids to 10% of our total calorie intake, while the American Heart Association favors a greater restriction, to just 7% of total calories. High intakes of most saturated fatty acids are linked to high levels of LDL (low-density lipoproteins), or "bad cholesterol," and reduced insulin sensitivity. However, even good sources of healthy fats (like nuts and salmon) may contain some saturated fatty acids, which is why they cannot be eliminated completely. Saturated fats are mostly those that are solid at room temperature (like the drippings that have cooled from a fatty piece of meat).

Trans fats are another category of fats. They are created in a process called hydrogenation, usually done to increase the shelf life of processed foods. This process creates both saturated and trans fats, but the ones that remain unsaturated in the process are changed in terms of their chemical structure. These fats that remain unsaturated are termed "trans fats" and are health-damaging. According to the NIH, these trans fats contribute to insulin resistance.[11] Additionally, these fats can raise LDL and also lower HDL cholesterol or "good cholesterol." These reasons are why the American Heart Association recommends that we keep our trans fatty acid intake to less than 1% of total calories consumed. Unfortunately, identifying trans fats in the American diet can be tricky. They are sometimes disguised under names such as "partially hydrogenated oil." Additionally, the law allows manufacturers to claim zero trans fats as long as a single serving contains no more than 0.49 grams.

The last category of fats are called unsaturated fats. WHO recommends that fats consumed by everyone two years of age or older should be primarily unsaturated fatty acids, with no more than 10% of total energy intake coming from them.[12] There are two types of unsaturated fats: monounsaturated and polyunsaturated. They both improve blood cholesterol levels and insulin sensitivity when they replace saturated and trans fats. Monounsaturated fats include sources like peanut, canola, and olive oils. Food sources for monounsaturated fats include nuts, seeds, olives, and avocados.

Polyunsaturated fats come in several types and have different roles in the body. Examples of these polyunsaturated fats types include Omega-3 and Omega-6 fatty acids. Omega-3 fatty acids include ALA (alpha linoleic acid), which your body is not able to create and needs through a healthy diet. From ALA, the body converts it into EPA and

DHA (both of which can be derived from various types of fish). Omega-6 fatty acids include LA (linoleic acid), another polyunsaturated fat that has to be acquired through the diet. Many cooking oils (such as corn, sunflower, safflower, and sesame) have Omega-6 fatty acids, in addition to many types of seeds (Brazil nuts, pecans, and pine nuts).

Fats, along with carbohydrates, is another macronutrient category that has been demonized at times in our American diet. In the 1980s and 1990s—when the low-fat approach became an overarching ideology promoted by physicians, the federal government, the food industry, and the popular health media—my household became a campaign for everything "fat free." My refrigerator through middle school and high school was stocked with fat-free dairy products, some of which seemed to never melt when being heated (like the fat-free cheese slices that were wrapped in plastic).

My mother treated fat like it was the devil, doing everything possible to make sure she and her family didn't go near it. Every once in a while she'd allow herself an egg for breakfast, but when making an omelet, she would have an egg-white only one cooked in fat-free margarine. The crazy thing is that the rest of our refrigerator and our pantry were stocked with processed and high-glycemic foods that were much more unhealthy for us than an extra egg or two, in lieu of nutrient-dense, wholesome foods.

I've learned over the years, and through my own education and experience, that all of the macronutrients are important. There isn't any benefit from demonizing one type of food over another or eliminating it altogether. Food types shouldn't be feared but rather chosen wisely when practicing a healthy diet. The important thing when distributing your daily amounts of each macronutrient into your diet is making sure you don't exceed your daily caloric needs (TDEE). This is the point where you gain unnecessary body fat. Additionally, finding a healthy distribution of each macronutrient is key to ensuring that you are satiated throughout the day and getting all of the macronutrients (and micronutrients) that you need. You can also enjoy some of your nutritional splurges when you understand what, and how much, of each macronutrient you're consuming.

SUMMARY

If you've finished reading this chapter and have taken the time to understand the basic principles of nutrition and fitness as it relates to energy balance and macronutrients, you've already taken the first step to reaching your goals! You will now be able to apply your knowledge in the following chapters, to create your own individualized nutrition and fitness plan with the ReShapeHER program and reach your goals **in as little as 4-6 weeks!**

In the following chapter, you will learn how to identify and avoid common pitfalls that mothers make when it comes to nutrition and fitness. With your knowledge of the basic principles of nutrition and fitness, complemented with the ReShapeHER Program, as well as understanding how to avoid these common pitfalls, you will be on your way to achieving your body composition goals.

CHAPTER 4 CLIFF NOTES

- "Energy Balance" (in terms of calorie storage or expenditure) is critical to understand when it comes to fitness outcomes. Exercise and nutritional tracking is an essential component of this.
- There is not a calorie that doesn't matter, in that the body is doing one of two things with them—storing them (resulting in fat loss unless they are eventually expended) or dealing with a deficit (resulting in fat loss over time).
- Your total daily energy expenditure (TDEE) over the course of a day is actually composed of four different values that make up its 100%. The 20% that you can control, consists of your NEAT (unplanned exercise) and your EAT (planned exercise). Your unplanned exercise actually makes up the majority of this percentage (15%) and can be manipulated based on the number of movements you make over time.

TDEE

REE*	70% of TDEE (resting energy expenditure)
NEAT	15% of TDEE (unplanned exercise)
TEF*	10% of TDEE (thermal effects of food)
EAT	5% of TDEE (planned exercise—resistance training and cardio)
TDEE	100%

**REE and TEF make up 80% of TDEE (equals a mother's BMI value)*

- A "diet", (in which you would consume fewer calories will enable the body to have less of an ability to store) creates an environment for fat loss, but should be practiced infrequently and only until your fat loss goals are achieved, as to avoid muscle loss and metabolic adaptation over time.

- When a lower body weight is achieved through dieting, it is critical to recalculate your TDEE, as this value will lower as body weight does. This will in turn, affect the values that make up your TDEE (REE, NEAT, TEF and EAT).
- Muscle mass, body fat mass, bone, and water, all contribute to your overall scale weight. These values can vary from day-to-day, and fluctuate based on a number of factors.
- In order to determine true body fat loss or gain, it is essential for a successful fitness plan to include body composition analysis as the primary tool used to determine progress in lieu of the common scale.
- Understanding the three macronutrients (proteins, carbohydrates and fats), and the role they serve in your diet, is the key to knowing what types (and how much) of foods, you should consume for fitness success.
- The AMDR recommendations for the three macronutrients are as follows: proteins at 10–35% per day, carbohydrates at 45–65% per day and fats at less than 20–35% for women ages 19 years and older.
- All macronutrients serve an important role in the body and no particular one should be demonized.

NOTES

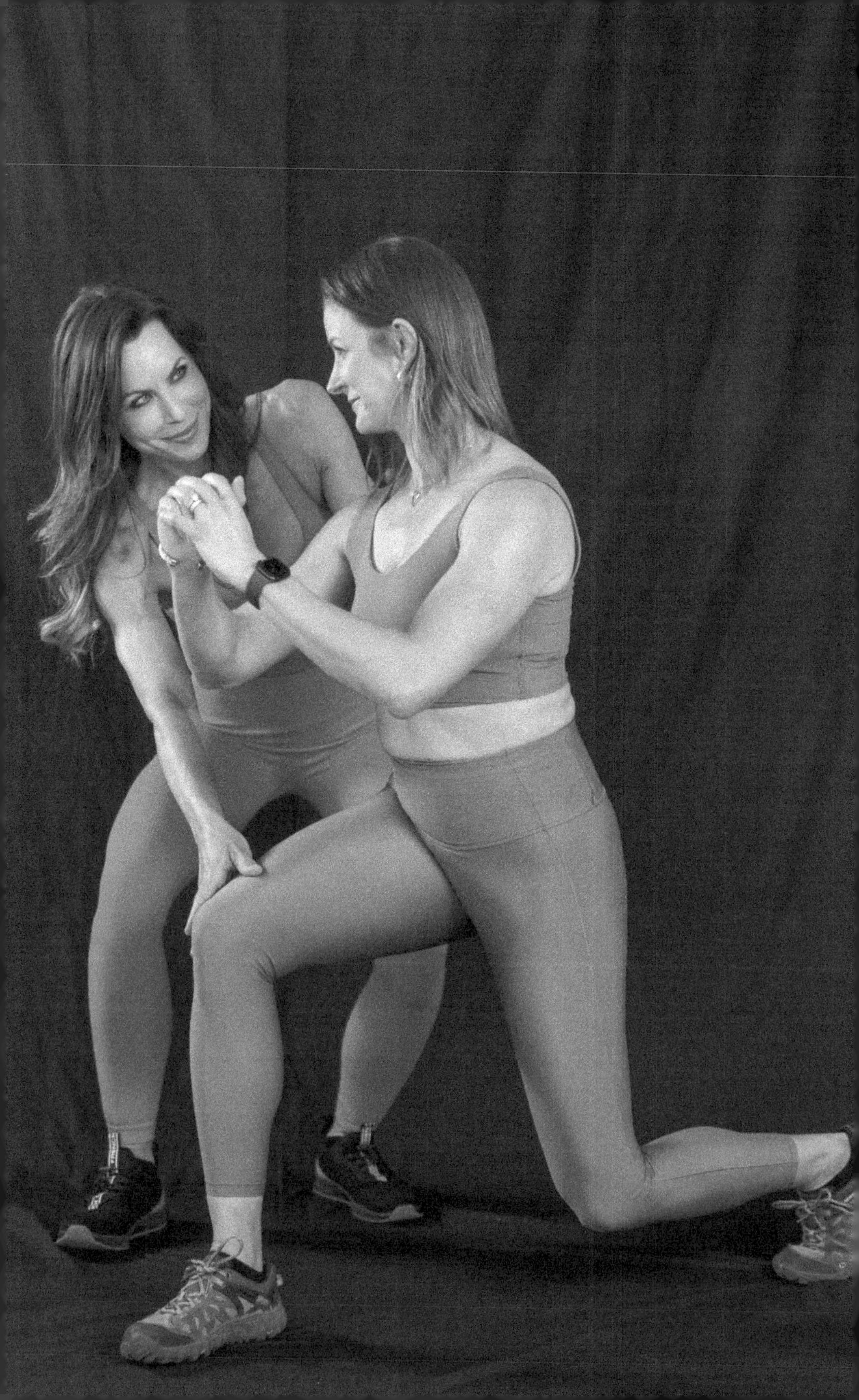

5

The Biggest Fitness Pitfalls Mothers Fall Prey To

THEY SAY THAT FAILURE CAN actually be one of our greatest learning lessons. I would have to agree. However, the greatest part of these lessons can only be found if we can identify the areas we fell off track. Only from this perspective, can we successfully implement new ideas, new approaches and new strategies to bring us success. This is the main focus of this chapter—to identify the areas that haven't brought mothers success and how these can be avoided with the ReShapeHER Fitness program.

Our society can unfortunately be a great breeding ground for these pitfalls, allowing many mothers to fall into their trap, oftentimes in more areas than one. It is absolutely critical that as mothers we don't fall prey to this and become "habitual offenders" to these repetitive cycles of less-than-optimal behavior. We can avoid getting caught up in these snares through continued nutrition and fitness education. So keep reading to gain knowledge on how you can avoid these common pitfalls!

Pitfall #1 – The Poor Diet

Being a busy mom can make it hard to eat our required macronutrient portions during snacks and mealtimes. Good food sources that contain macronutrients like protein and fiber, aren't usually ones that are packed and prepared, easy for us to grab which help contribute to our overall satiety and lend to our overall over-consumption of calories. We also tend to spend the least amount of time focused on our nutritional needs in lieu of our children's. We may find ourselves even eating their leftovers to replace a meal that we would have otherwise had. Most of the convenient snacks that are easy to consume with busy schedules, tend to be ones that are high in carbohydrates and fat. Food companies are also aware that this combination of macronutrients allows the taste of foods to be superior to others as well, driving us to consume them for these reasons in addition to their convenience.

A large part of why we fail to reach our goals simply comes down to a lack of understanding food values and how much of each food contributes to our overall protein requirements. Take peanut butter, for example. This is a food that is assumed to be high in protein; however, it consists of mostly fat, as two tablespoons have a whopping 250 calories and only eight grams of protein yet double that amount in fat. (This is a tough one to admit, considering peanut butter is one of my favorite foods!). Peanut butter can still be successfully included in a mother's diet, however, this is done by paying attention to serving sizes and with other foods that have higher protein and carbohydrate values to ensure a mother is eating a balanced diet and staying within her daily calories.

In addition to the overconsumption of non-nutritious convenient foods and our lack of understanding of food values, lies the fact that as mothers, we often don't make our diet a priority. Think about the last time you prepared dinner for the family. . . were you mindful of making sure you had a balanced portion of protein, carbohydrates and fats? Or, did you just eat what sounded good for everyone else? Did your snacks earlier in the day consist of leftover foods your kids didn't eat or foods that were chosen for convenience over their wholesome value? When we ask ourselves these questions, we can begin to realize how much we haven't prioritized our own needs in terms of meeting our nutritional goals as mothers.

As I discussed in the previous chapter, protein is the macronutrient that provides us the building blocks to support and grow lean muscle tissue. Without an adequate amount, we not only leave our bodies without support for a healthy body composition, but also leave it at risk for developing many health issues, such as a lowered immune system and an increase in bone fractures to name a few. According to the American Bone Health and Osteoporosis Foundation (BHOF), "women are far more likely to have a fracture than men, in fact, one in two women over the age of 50 will have a fracture in her lifetime." This organization states that this is because women's bones, even at their best (ages 25–30), are generally smaller and less dense than men's bones.[13] With that said, I'm sure we would all agree that women need to be making their protein requirements a priority, simply because we are genetically more at risk for these types of health detriments. This is one of the greatest areas of nutritional education that needs to be supported for all women.

In the following chapter, I discuss why the ReShapeHER program supports Nutritional tracking, and how through this practice, a mother can receive a priceless education on how to understand her individual requirements and portion sizes through this practice. Through the experience of nutritional tracking, I'll help a mother understand how she'll be able to control her outcomes and know how to maintain her ideal body composition over a short period of time!

Pitfall #2 – The Yo-Yo Diet

I've discussed how cliche the word "diet" has become in our society, making us women feel like we constantly need to be practicing one. In lieu of thinking of "diet" in terms of focusing on our overall nutrition, we equate it to practicing a restrictive intake of any form of food with our all-or-nothing, modern-day approaches, versus considering what it is that we are restricting.

Crash diets have become the rage, with a romanticized idea of how they'll ultimately result in bringing us the fitness results we are looking for. According to a *Women's Health* magazine article, Benjamin Gardner (a health research psychologist at King's College London, specializing in behavioral change and habit formation) states that "apart from making you feel like you're getting a clean break from your bad behaviors, many of us tend to be overly confident about our ability to stick with plans that aren't completely sustainable." He also states that "trying to maintain high levels of effort to control our diet and exercise can deplete our willpower." He further explains why this leads to further relapses, and thus, the yo-yo cycle of dieting.[14]

This yo-yo dieting is one of the biggest pitfalls that derails us women in achieving our fitness goals. Besides leading to us feeling like failures when our willpower can't keep up with our restrictive practices, there are many other metabolic reasons as to why this type of practice makes a negative contribution to our efforts.

Yo-yo dieting is a result of desperate attempts we make to restrict our overall calories in order to lose weight. As a result of this aggressive restriction, we fail in our attempts to keep any weight loss in the long term, as this practice can simply not be sustained. Therefore, our yo-yo dieting attempts result in us gaining back the weight that we lost, encouraging us to make more attempts at trying to lose this weight that was gained back. What results is an undulating cycle that brings us away from, and back to, our weight loss starting points (with negative impacts on our overall health).

These unsuccessful attempts at our diet mimic that of the back-and-forth movements of a yo-yo released from a starting point that it will inevitably return to. The calorie reductions that we are making not only reduce our daily calorie intake (TDEE) over time but also the intake of our overall macronutrients as a result. When we do this, we naturally consume less of each macronutrient.

If we aren't paying special attention to the balance of each macronutrient that we're consuming, we could lend ourselves to not consuming enough of one or more of them, resulting in the body not having enough of them to carry out its necessary functions. For example, restricting our overall calories could result in us not consuming enough protein, resulting in us losing previous lean muscle tissue that we worked so hard to maintain or grow. This muscle loss would result in not only a less favorable body composition but also lead to other risks to our bodies. These risks could include things such as a possible weakened immune system, inflammation, poor hair and skin, brittle nails, irregular periods, high blood pressure, weakened bones, and risks of bone fractures.

Considering women are already at risk for bone loss as we age, reducing our protein requirements is certainly something that doesn't contribute to our overall health. Outside of protein alone, if we aren't consuming enough carbohydrates and fats, this can also result in less-than-optimal health results. It is critical that women consume enough fats to support hormonal health. If we don't consume enough, this could lead to many health detriments, such as mood changes and hormonal imbalances. Not consuming enough carbohydrates can lead to possible weakness, fatigue, hypoglycemia, and many other health risks.

In addition to the risks that are associated with not consuming enough of each macronutrient, yo-yo dieting puts women at risk for less optimal body composition changes. With a decrease in muscle tissue, the body compensates for this by filling the void with body fat over time. Therefore, with a decrease in lean muscle tissue and an increase in body fat, this changes a woman's body composition over time, resulting in raising her overall BMI and body fat percentage. Along with these body composition changes, she also makes negative contributions to her overall metabolism due to this muscle loss, in addition to driving her body to make adaptive changes.

When a woman drives down her daily calories and forces her body to lose weight (as this scale weight isn't indicative of what she lost in terms of muscle or body fat), she also drives the body's desire to compensate for these aggressive changes. Metabolic adaptation occurs when the body fights to keep its weight steady and is able to "adapt" and function in conditions in which our energy consumption is lower, as it is able to lower our metabolism in order to achieve this. What many women fail to realize in general is that with a decrease in weight, this also decreases her overall daily calories demand. This decrease in daily calorie requirement, combined with the body's ability to make adaptations to maintain its weight at lower energy levels by decreasing its metabolism, is what makes this type of dieting an ultimate failure in terms of maintaining overall fitness success.

Maintaining this lower weight and trying to overcome the body's successful ability to adapt is what results in women's unsuccessful attempts at this type of dieting, and also what lures them into the trap of this type of dieting. Although these drastic attempts may lend results in the beginning, they are unrealistic to maintain over time. More importantly to understand is that they also serve as detrimental to a woman's overall health and fitness goals. Fitness experts understand this process, which is why they will allow their bodies "diet breaks" in order to ward off this adaptation and allow their bodies time to recover from it and respond to their future diet attempts. They spend this time not only recovering from this adaptation, but also working to reverse this natural phenomenon as they use the science of energy balance to drive up their calorie intake as high as possible, without sacrificing their body compensation.

This process can be very complicated and highly individualized. It is an area that bodybuilders learn to become experts at, yet the general public struggles to grasp the most simple concepts. A large majority of our general public of women continue to practice this yo-yo dieting, not understanding how this negative practice contributes to their long-term health and fitness outcomes.

Yo-yo dieting and the metabolic adaptation it creates in terms of how it affects our body composition isn't the only negative contribution it makes in terms of our fitness. This type of dieting also creates a large amount of stress on the female body. Constant dieting can trigger an increase in stress hormones, cortisol specifically, that leads to an increase in visceral fat. These increases in stress hormones can wreak havoc on a female body, leading to inflammation, amenorrhea, poor sleep, mood changes, etc. When these hormones are imbalanced, it may take a woman many months, even years, to correct. Personally, I've experienced many times in which my hormones were imbalanced, derailing me from my fitness goals and leaving me with a shitload of symptoms to manage. I used to put the blame on these occurrences as par for the course to being a woman, when in fact it was my constant yo-yo dieting that was to blame. Being a woman can be hard enough with our monthly hormonal fluctuations we experience each month, without adding an additional stressor to these cyclical changes.

I discuss in Chapter 7, how the ReShapeHER program can help a mother control her dietary efforts with a "seasonal" approach. By taking this seasonal approach, I'll explain how she can ultimately learn how she can control her nutritional intake, and by doing this, how she can avoid unhealthy adaptations and quickly achieve the body composition she desires!

Pitfall #3 – Muscle Loss

When we only dedicate our fitness efforts with movements that only contribute to our calorie output alone, our efforts become one-dimensional as we are simply just managing our energy balance. The other part of our planned exercise (EAT) that we are failing to have a benefit from, resistance training, allows us to not only manage our energy balance but also helps to build our muscle tissue, which allows us to achieve our best body composition. Additionally, this muscle tissue allows us to protect our organs and joints, maintain a healthy bone density and support a healthy metabolism.

Fitness programs that are void of resistance training, don't allow for mothers to achieve muscle maintenance or growth. When you combine this with the practices of yo-yo dieting, this results in an actual reduction of muscle tissue on a mother's body over time. As a result, this further drives a woman even closer to a less-than-optimal body composition. And to make matters worse, if her cardiovascular efforts decrease after these body composition changes and she isn't able to contribute as much to her caloric output, she will end up gaining body fat and her body composition will be even less desirable.

I discuss in Chapter 9 how a mother can focus her resistance training efforts with specific compound and isolation lifts. Additionally, I will discuss how along with a healthy diet, the ReShapeHER 3-Day or 5-Day Fitness Plans can bring her body quick results and help her successfully attack common problem areas: abdominals, glutes, thighs, hamstrings, as well as her upper body. In this chapter, a mother can say goodbye to the all-too-common "muffin top", "banana roll", "saddlebags" and "bat wings"!

Pitfall #4 – Too Much Planned Cardio

As mothers, sometimes we can fall victim to being so hyper-focused on body fat loss and its contribution to our body composition that we only perform exercises that allow us to make changes in this area. We fail to consider the other half of the body composition equation—our muscle composition. In doing this, we have been notorious for having a gym membership to monopolize the treadmill and other cardiovascular machines. We have become the reason why the term "cardio bunny" is in the urban dictionary, as we've dedicated hours on end to devote as much time to our caloric output to make a dent in our body fat.

Of course, as much as cardiovascular activities are good for our cardio health, some would argue that this benefit hasn't been the motive for our efforts. In fact, if we were worried about our overall health, we wouldn't have avoided resistance training, in lieu of cardio alone, for our overall fitness health. With our mistake of focusing too much on planned cardio alone, we may have put ourselves at risk for muscle loss in lieu of muscle gain, negating our efforts to achieve our ideal body composition.

In Chapter 10, I discuss how a mother can use her unplanned cardio (NEAT) in the ReShapeHER Fitness program, as a secret weapon in driving up her overall calorie expenditure. Through her efforts, she will be able to make the best use of her time in working towards achieving the body composition of her dreams in little time!

By understanding these four pitfalls that many mothers make when it comes to fitness, you can see why it is that many of us women fail to reach our fitness goals. Whether they may be one mistake out of the four or all of them collectively, they can potentially result in not only failed fitness attempts but also health-related risks. It is critical that we continue seeking fitness education as mothers, to ensure we aren't making these mistakes and contributing to helping others do the same.

It is my personal goal and mission to educate mothers through this book, in order to drive this fitness education and to stop them from being victims to these pitfalls that have led them to fail to reach their fitness goals. Additionally, through the ReShapeHER Program, I provide all mothers with an obtainable outline that avoids all four of these detrimental pitfalls and leads them to fitness success. It is my hope that one day, these common pitfalls will be lost in history through the practice of this program.

CHAPTER 5 CLIFF NOTES

- There are four major pitfalls mothers fall prey to, when it comes to fitness: The Poor Diet, The Yo-Yo Diet, Muscle Loss and Too Much Cardio.
- Overconsumption of non-nutritious convenient foods, our lack of understanding of food values and not making our diet a priority are areas where mothers fall prey to a poor diet.
- A decrease in our daily calorie intake (TDEE), combined with the body's ability to make adaptations to maintain its weight at lower energy levels by decreasing its metabolism, in addition to the stress it places on the female body, is what makes the Yo-Yo dieting pitfall an ultimate failure for mothers when it comes to their fitness.
- Mothers can fall into the pitfall of muscle loss, when they don't support their muscle with enough calories (too much restriction over time), the right types of calories (adhering to an adequate amount of protein in their diet) and not practicing Resistance training in their fitness plan.
- Mothers can fall prey to doing an excessive amount of cardio in their fitness plan, putting themselves at risk for muscle loss in lieu of muscle gain and negating their efforts to achieve an ideal body composition.

NOTES

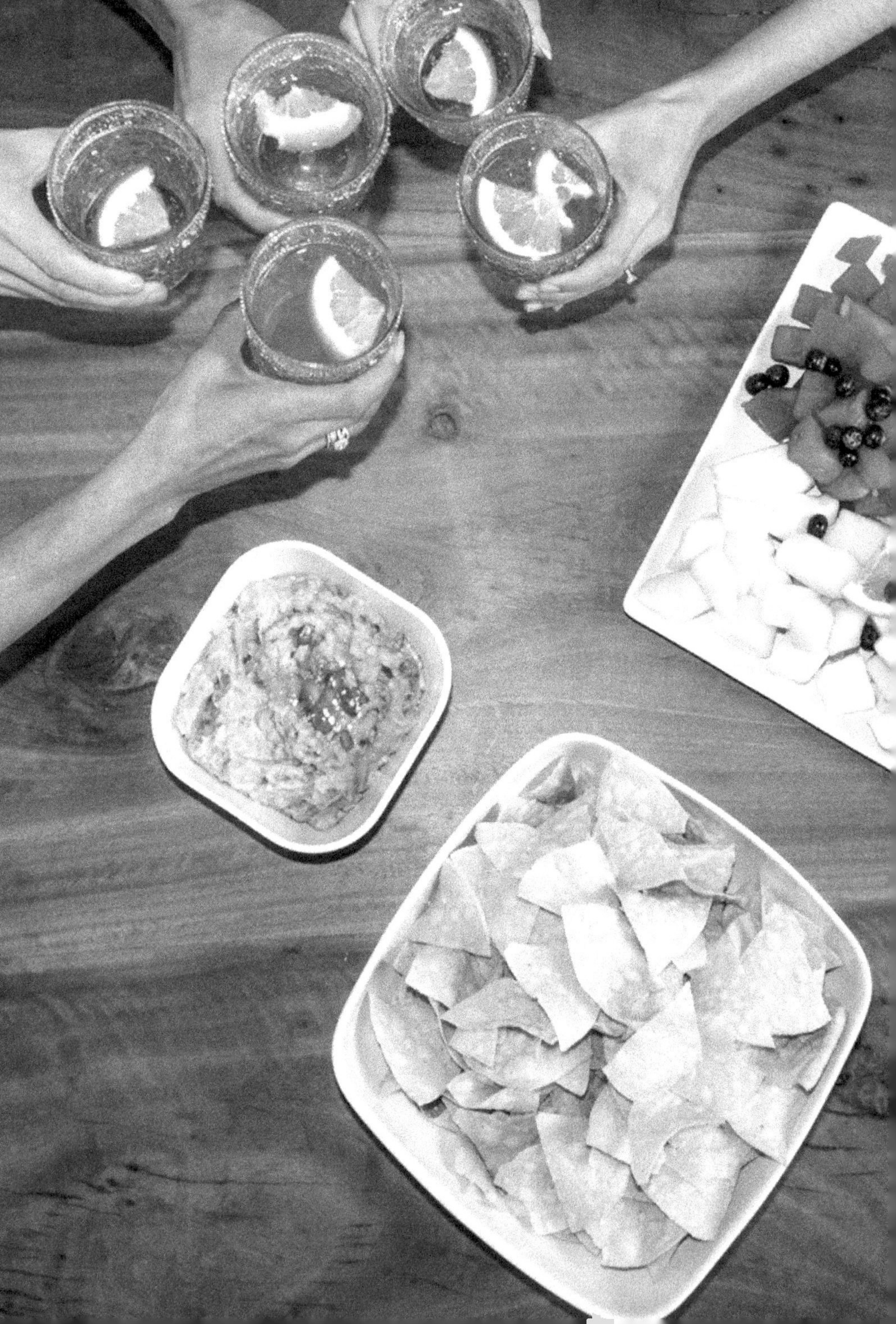

6

Combating Pitfall #1

—The Poor Diet

ARE YOU READY TO START applying your nutrition and fitness understanding to Pitfall #1, "The Poor Diet?" Remember, only through the process of identifying the decisions that led to this pitfall and forming a strategy that avoids it, can we move beyond this trap. In this chapter, I will simplify the process of calculating two values that will lead you to success when it comes to your diet: your **Daily Calories** and **Macronutrient values**. With that said, there is some reading involved on your part, to make sure you have the education you need to be successful. This chapter may start out a little didactic, but at the end of each section, there is a video you can simply "Click", and it will give you the easiest way you can apply the information you've learned in this chapter. At the end of this chapter, you will know how to successfully avoid the trap of "The Poor Diet"!

As the old saying goes, "Abs are built in the kitchen." It is true that body composition results can be achieved by knowing what, and how much, of the right foods contribute to our fitness success. Once I began the practice of diligently tracking my food specifically to my goals, I was able to have a much clearer understanding of how I could accomplish my nutritional goals in a short period of time. With my newfound knowledge of food and energy balance, I realized I had total control of my fitness outcomes. I began to realize that without this knowledge, mothers fall short of achieving what they want with their nutrition and overall fitness.

Because food labeling wasn't required until the late 1990s and became much more specific after 2016, I'm certain that this lack of important information is the reason why so many people in general don't have an idea of what they're eating and how to track their nutrition. When I think about how important this nutritional education is, in that it serves as the very backbone to ensuring someone has a successful diet that allows them to reach their health and fitness goals, it floors me that we don't teach this in our educational system. The frustration I feel when I think about how far we are behind the eight ball with teaching this information, it is often hard to contain my emotions.

Most of our teachers are not equipped as health and fitness educators. The foods that are being provided at schools are also a reflection of this lack of education. Couple all of this with coming out of a recent pandemic that shifted our lives more indoors with a lesser amount of required movement and the rising costs of foods (especially healthier ones) due to inflation, and we are not exactly set up for health and fitness success. Despite all of this, we can do better! There is a great opportunity for us mothers to come together and insist on better nutritional education for not only ourselves but also for our children right now!

The caveat to our modern-day society is that although we have a lot of tracking tools at our disposal, there isn't a lot of education and awareness surrounding them. The problem with these devices that track our movements, and especially the ones that are built into the machines we may see at our local gyms (like the treadmills), is that they are based on general calculations and lack specificity to an individual (like their body composition data). This often lends us to making over assumptions of how many calories we are burning during a workout. According to Stanford Medicine in their article that addresses fitness activity trackers, none of the seven devices in their study measured energy expenditure accurately. The study found that even the most accurate device was off by an average of 27%. The least accurate was off by 93%.[15] This is the reason why it's important for a mother to invest in a personalized tracker that provides more specificity to her own body and movements, and sets a daily movement goal to ensure that she's contributing successfully to her calorie expenditure.

Other tools such as the nutritional tracking applications are available that can help a mother determine her overall calories per day (TDEE). These applications can provide incredible insight into a mother's diet, in terms of not only understanding how much she should consume each day, but also how she achieves this goal over time and ways to make improvements with this data. These applications take the headache out of helping a mother determine not only her daily calories, but can also break down her macronutrient percentages and also provide her a target daily calorie value if she'd like to lose or gain weight. There are also many other types of functionalities within these applications, such as the ability to track body weight, track recipes, join social groups, etc. The downside of these nutritional tracking tools is that there is always room for human error when it comes to their associated food databases. According to the *Journal of Medical Internet Research*, in their dietary analysis of the MyFitnessPal app, although this app served accurately and efficiently for total energy intake, macronutrients, sugar, and fiber, it did not for cholesterol and sodium.[16] In addition to the possibility of inaccuracies with nutritional values, activity multipliers can be confusing as a mother may enter a level of activity that she doesn't fulfill on a daily basis. Despite these nutritional tracking inaccuracies, I would argue that the pros of these tools far outweigh the cons when it comes to understanding how to track one's nutrition and truly understand the value of the foods that are being consumed. If we understand the science behind how and why we track (that you'll learn in this book), these applications can be incredibly useful when we are able to obtain more precise information on our specific variables, as they relate to our nutritional requirements.

THE IMPORTANCE OF CALCULATING YOUR TOTAL DAILY ENERGY EXPENDITURE (TDEE)

My history of calorie tracking started in my early adult life, when I started learning that there was an energy weight attached to the foods that I was eating. I started paying attention to labels (only in terms of calories) at the turn of the 21st century, when this type of information was being provided on foods. I learned to avoid foods that were "higher" in calories and favor ones that were less. I even experienced weight loss by making these choices, although I went by scale weight alone, as my education of body composition took place much later in my fitness journey.

I was a cardio "queen" and spent hours running on treadmills in the gym, especially if I knew I had over-consumed these calorie-laden foods and needed to combat the weight gain I made with them. I never took the time, nor did I have the education, to understand what these calories were made up of. It was only much later in my life that I understood how these calories I was consuming were distributed and broken down into their macronutrient components. Because of this lack of nutritional information I lacked earlier in my life, I spent many years fueling my body (although athletic) with a poor diet, which is why I failed to reach my ultimate fitness potential.

Before I get into the nuts and bolts of calorie calculating, it is critical to understand one's daily caloric limit (TDEE; total daily energy expenditure). This number will represent the number of calories (in terms of energy) your body needs to maintain itself. A lower TDEE per day (fewer calories consumed through diet or fewer calories as a result of higher calorie outputs contributed through exercise/movement) results in body weight loss. A higher TDEE (more calories consumed through diet or more calories as a result of lower calorie outputs contributed through exercise/movement) results in body weight gain. *There is NO WAY around the truth that CALORIES ARE KING (or in our case, QUEEN!)*

What you consume in terms of your diet plays the biggest part in reaching or not reaching your TDEE. This is why understanding how much food in terms of calories you can eat each day, as well as the amounts of macronutrients you'll need that these foods are made of (these are discussed in the next section), is critical when you want to reach your fitness goals.

Value #1—How To Calculate Your Daily Calories (TDEE)

Before calculating your TDEE, a mother must understand what goes into the calculations. It is critical to remember that these are only calculations, so the numbers they provide are generalizations, as they don't take into consideration a mother's body composition, which would provide more data than just age, height, and weight. Therefore, it's critical to remember that individual responses may vary when it comes to a set TDEE, which is why it's critical to re-calculate these values every 2–4 weeks to allow for adjustments to reach one's fitness goals.

Also, the primary value you calculate is your BMR (basal metabolic rate). Your BMR is basically the minimum amount of calories that your body needs to perform necessary functions (like pumping blood, digesting food, etc.). This value alone is 70% of your TDEE! So basically, your body's ability just to exist requires this amount of your overall daily caloric consumption... wild, I know.

When your BMR is combined with your thermal effects of food (in other words, the calories burned just metabolizing your food; TEF), you are already at 80% of your TDEE. The remaining 20% make up your overall daily movements in terms of your planned exercise (EAT) and your unplanned exercise (NEAT). These exercises are considered through the activity multipliers that are given with the below suggested calculations. So, in summary, 100% of your TDEE is made up of 70% BMR, 10% TEF, 15% NEAT, and 5% EEE.

I will entertain those of you who like to do Math problems below (otherwise, keep reading to find out your TDEE and macronutrient values the easy way with the ReShapeHER Video!)

When you calculate your BMR, you will be multiplying it by an activity factor that represents the average amount of daily activity you achieve. According to Medscape, a comparative study of four predictive equations found that the Mifflin-St Jeor equation (introduced in 1990) is more likely than the other equations to predict BMR within 10% of that measured.[17] However, the Katch-McArdle formula can be more accurate for people who are leaner and know their body fat percentages (as this is considered more accurate than other formulas based on total body weight alone). However, there are very few people who are aware of their body fat; therefore, the Mifflin-St Jeor equation is one that is the tried and true staple for most.

Below is how you calculate your BMR with the Mifflin-St Jeor formula:

FEMALES: {10 x Weight (kg)} + {6.25 x height (cm)} – {5 x age (years)} – 161

MALES: {10 x weight (kg)} + {6.25 x height (cm)} – {5 x age (years)} + 5

You will then multiply your result from above, by your following activity level:

Sedentary: x 1.2
Lightly active: x 1.375
Moderately active: x 1.55
Active: x 1.725
Very active: x 1.9

For example, for a 30-year-old female weighing 150 pounds and standing five-foot-eight with a moderate activity level, the following would be her BMR calculation:

{10 x 68.18 8kg} + {6.25 x 172.72 cm} – {5 x 30} – 161

681.80 + 1,079.50 – 150 – 161 = 1,450.30 BMR

Because this female has a moderate activity level, her BMR would be multiplied by an activity factor of 1.55 to figure out her overall TDEE (total daily energy expenditure):

1,450.30 x 1.55 = 2,247.965 TDEE

So for this particular female, she has a BMR of 1,450.30, but due to her activity level, she has an overall calorie allotment of 2,247.965 calories per day (TDEE). Based on this TDEE, she can then calculate how many of each macronutrient that should make up this TDEE in order to ensure that she reaches her fitness goals (this is discussed in the next section).

It is important to note that with fluctuating weight changes, it is important to adjust one's TDEE every 2–4 weeks!

How the ReshapeHER Program Helps You Understand How to Calculate Your TDEE With One Simple Click!

Watch this video to find out how!

**Note: these macronutrient values will fluctuate up and down as TDEE values do. Therefore, adjustments to TDEE will also reflect adjustments to macronutrient values.*

WHY MACRONUTRIENTS NEED TO BE CONSIDERED WITH YOUR TDEE

I discussed in the above ReShapeHER video, how understanding how to calculate your daily calories allows you to obtain the first steps in controlling the nutritional part of your fitness plan as well as your fitness outcomes. In my opinion, this process is something every woman should know how to do in their life, because if they did, we would have a much greater understanding of food values and how this applies to achieving our fitness goals.

However, calorie tracking won't lead you to your fitness goals alone. The second step is understanding the three macronutrients that make up these calories. Knowing how to successfully calculate and balance these three macronutrients, allows you to consume their amounts that support our necessary bodily functions that promote good health and can lead all of us mothers to achieving the body composition we desire.

Although you already have the suggested values for macronutrients from the video, it's imperative that you continue reading, to understand why the ReShapeHER program suggests these values!

Our total daily energy expenditure (TDEE), which we often think of in terms of the daily calories our body burns, determines how much of all three macronutrients we can consume. Macronutrients are the nutrients we need in order for our bodies to perform the various functions they need in order to survive. These macronutrients are made up of proteins, carbohydrates, and fats. The type of balance we create with all three of these macronutrients, as well as how well we stay within our daily calories for a healthy body weight, is what provides us with or without a healthy diet. This balance is highly individualized and requires a solid nutritional plan.

Should we adjust our TDEE, our macronutrients would then need to be adjusted (as all three make up our daily calories). Conversely, should we choose to adjust the value of one of our macronutrients, the other two would also have to be adjusted, as all three of them equal our overall TDEE. Daily calorie adjustments are made if we choose to increase or decrease our energy balance, resulting in us burning fewer or more calories per day. Along with these adjustments, this in turn affects the values of the macronutrients that make up our overall daily calories.

Knowing that each macronutrient plays a specific role in bodily functions, and making adjustments to them, can help us achieve our fitness goals. For example, because protein can contribute to muscle maintenance and growth, consuming recommended protein values can allow us to achieve this and contribute to overall better body composition. Ensuring that we have an ample amount of protein in our diet is critical to ensure that we are able to achieve this healthy composition and maintain it, which is why it is important to prioritize protein when it comes to calculating and/or adjusting one's macronutrient values.

Carbohydrates and fats, although not as important for muscle development but important in terms of being consumed for other bodily functions at recommended levels, also help us achieve our fitness goals. Every macronutrient plays its part in ensuring that we achieve a healthy diet. If a woman chooses to eat a higher-protein diet that is less in carbs and higher in fat, it doesn't mean she can't achieve optimal fitness outcomes more than a woman who chooses to have a higher-protein diet that is higher in carbs and lower in fat. Fitness outcomes all come down to individualized responses. However, the one thing that should remain a commonality with any woman is to ensure that she's prioritizing protein to support her lean muscle tissue. Fats and carbohydrates (both important and should be consumed, at the least, by their minimal recommendations) can be interchangeable when it comes to being calculated after protein values have been determined.

When it comes to understanding the fitness values I'm discussing, one might ask, "What's the most important thing... knowing your TDEE per day or your macronutrient values that make up your TDEE?" Here's the answer: Knowing your daily TDEE, because the principles of energy balance always reign supreme. *Remember, CALORIES ARE QUEEN!* However, both are incredibly important.

Although energy balance (daily calories) reigns supreme no matter what you eat, you will gain with a calorie surplus and lose with a calorie deficit. The nutritional content of what you're consuming (as determined by your macros) will ultimately determine your health outcomes. If you ate donuts for a month and stayed under your required TDEE, you would lose weight but what would your health look like? I think you can answer that question.

Additionally, each macronutrient provides the body with different benefits. Protein is essential for developing healthy muscles, and there's not much protein in a standard donut. If you ate donuts for a straight month, do you think your body would have the basic protein requirements it would need to develop healthy muscle tissue? You could guess the answer, but if you successfully tracked this diet, you would know that the answer to this is no. A donut is composed of mostly low-glycemic carbohydrates and saturated fat. You could certainly lose weight if you ate under your TDEE for a month with calories coming from donuts; however, you would also lose precious muscle tissue in the process.

Due to this muscle tissue loss, your body composition would change as you would have less muscle to contribute to your overall lean mass weight. If you gained weight at a future date with increasing calories over your TDEE, you would certainly have a higher body fat percentage, as you gained in addition to having muscle loss. So you can see, just knowing your TDEE and staying within this value doesn't provide you with all of the necessary tools to have a healthy diet. It is absolutely essential to eat a balanced diet with all three macronutrients, and stay within one's TDEE, in order to guarantee a healthy diet.

It is important to note that when tracking one's nutritional values, one person cannot compare their value to someone else's. Two people of the exact same scale weight but different body compositions can vary in their calorie and macronutrient requirements. A pregnant or lactating female would have much different requirements than a young female who isn't in a reproductive state. Males and females in general often differ in their macronutrient requirements. The message is to NEVER COMPARE your values with that of someone else's. I've discussed why the game of comparison is futile in terms of aesthetics, and it certainly applies when it comes to each woman's nutritional requirements. Additionally, this is an area that is important to note when it comes to working with a fitness expert. If they are recommending a nutritional guideline that is similar to all of their clients, BEWARE!

Value #2—How to Calculate Your Macronutrients

Once you successfully calculate your TDEE, you can begin the process of calculating your daily requirement for each of your macronutrients. This can be accomplished by calculating these requirements on your own (as I'll discuss in this section), or by simply entering them into your nutritional tracker (the EASY way and explained in the video at the end of this section). As a general rule of thumb, and for your own nutritional education, it is important to read labels and understand how these values apply to your individual nutritional requirements. Additionally, understanding these values will also help you make good decisions when it comes to portion sizes when you don't have the labels readily available.

When it comes to calculating one's macronutrients, it is important to know that "not all calories are created equal!" This common saying is reflective of the fact that the calories each macronutrient contributes to a diet are different. (Carbohydrates contribute 4kcal/g, proteins contribute 4kcal/g, and fats 9kcal/g). Depending on the distribution of these macronutrients, they also result in different fitness outcomes when it comes to reaching our fitness goals (of which I discuss further in this book).

Macronutrient Calorie Values:

Protein	4 kcal/g
Carbohydrates	4 kcal/g
Fats	9 kcal/g

The one macronutrient that has a notably higher thermic effect is protein (when being compared to carbohydrates and fats). This higher thermic effect results in a greater energy expenditure when consumed. As a result, a diet higher in protein would possibly result in a greater calorie expenditure, as it directly affects a mother's TEF (thermal effects of food), therefore possibly raising her TDEE (overall daily calorie requirement). *This is the reason, along with their ability to contribute the most to muscle maintenance and growth, as well as to increase a mother's satiety, why the ReShapeHER program prioritizes protein first when it comes to nutritional tracking.* Additionally, this is also the reason why the prioritization of protein is essential when it comes to combating the pitfall of a mother having a poor diet that is too low in this macronutrient.

Given that most foods contain a combination of all three macronutrients, measuring a mother's total calories that are consumed (TDEE) is still the most accurate way to measure her overall energy intake. This is why the values of the macronutrients are benchmarked against her TDEE when they are calculated.

Let's review the three macronutrients again: protein, carbohydrates, and fats. However, before I do, I need to discuss the dichotomy that exists between the governmental recommendations surrounding macronutrients and those supported by the fitness industry. This is an area that needs to be called out and needs much further education and updating. When you compare the RDA requirements for macronutrients to that of the fitness industry, many would argue that the lower end of the RDA requirements are not set up for women to achieve their best body compositions. For example, the RDA recommendation for the average woman is to have her protein be a total of 10–35% of her total calories.

I explain in this chapter how it could be argued that the lower end of the RDA's AMDR percentage requirements, as they relate to protein, might keep a mother from reaching her fitness goals. The ReShapeHER program considers this possibility and provides a mother with a successful nutritional guide that is still within the RDA's recommended AMDR range. However, the ReShapeHER program suggests a mother consumes her protein per the RDA's higher-end recommendation, so she can reach her body composition and fitness goals. This program prioritizes the protein macronutrient, as it contains the building blocks for maintaining and growing lean muscle tissue, followed by carbohydrates and fats.

As you consider the importance of macronutrients (and their distribution) as part of your healthy diet, it is also important to consider the micronutrients (the smaller, chemical elements or substances required in trace amounts for growth and development) that each macronutrient provides. When you drill each macronutrient down further, you can learn to appreciate the smaller elements that make each one up and realize why it's important to have all three macronutrients as part of a healthy diet. These micronutrients consist of elements that are required by the body in varying quantities and orchestrate a range of physiological functions to maintain good health. They are divided into four groups: water-soluble vitamins, fat-soluble vitamins, macrominerals, and trace minerals. Deficiency in any of them can cause severe and even life-threatening conditions.

Ensuring we get enough micronutrients in their required amounts is the reason why we often take multivitamins and other supplements to support our diets. You can see why a diet that restricts an entire macronutrient group can possibly be a dangerous practice, not only in terms of eliminating the benefits a macronutrient provides, but also that of its micronutrients! This is the reason why the ReShapeHER program does not support cutting out any one particular macronutrient for a mother to achieve her health and fitness goals, nor suggests or supports any supplement to take the place of whole nutrition.

UNDERSTANDING YOUR PROTEIN VALUES

As you recall from a previous chapter, you learned that protein is absolutely essential for building muscle mass (lean body tissue). Foods that contain protein are oftentimes very healthy, unless they are paired with saturated fats (such as a lean cut of meat yet soaked in a copious amount of butter). I'll start with this macronutrient, as this is the one that I recommend setting a woman's goals for first, considering she'll want to maintain and support, or grow, healthy muscle tissue. The basic RDA recommended intake for protein is 0.8g/kg of body weight (older adults may need consumption around 1.2g/kg). The basic RDA recommended dosage at 0.75g/kg would result in 54.54g of protein required for a 150-pound female (81.65g for an older female).

The RDA also states that protein should account for 10–35% of total calories (according to its AMDR). If this female has a caloric intake requirement of 2,000 calories to maintain her weight and activity level, going by the lower end of the RDA's AMDR range for daily protein intake, it means this amount of protein would account for about 10% of her daily caloric intake (equaling approximately 50g of total protein).

The College of Sports Medicine and the International Society of Sports Nutrition recommend that physically active females consume 1.4–2g of protein per kg of body weight per day in order to allow for recovery from training and to promote the growth and maintenance of lean body mass.[18] This would equate to a range of 20–27% of her daily caloric intake. (The fitness industry, especially the bodybuilding world, would argue that it needs to be on the higher end of this range to support optimal muscle maintenance and growth). *Therefore, you can see where the differences lie when it comes to a woman's dietary recommendation for protein when it pertains to the lower end of the RDA's recommended AMDR range.*

An article by Health.com on protein deficiency states that "even though many people think the protein RDA is the recommended optimal intake, it's actually the minimum amount of protein necessary to prevent muscle loss. This means that most people need to take in more protein to maintain optimal health." The author also states that "people who are pregnant or breastfeeding, older adults, and those with medical conditions that increase protein needs like cancer also have greater protein requirements than the general population."[19]

The ReShapeHER program suggests a mother's protein intake at the higher end of the RDA's recommended AMDR percentage range for total overall protein consumption. This means that this program recommends that females set their overall protein intake to around 30% (give or take 5%) of overall total calories.

For the average female weighing 150 pounds and eating an average of 2,000 calories per day, this would equate to about 125–175 grams of protein per day. This would equal 600 calories of protein consumed per day (if consuming an optimal 150 grams), as you would divide the number of grams by four (as each gram of protein equates to four calories). The following calculation can be used to determine protein consumption:

Total calories per day x 25–35% = Total calories of protein recommended per day

Total calories of protein recommended per day ÷ 4 (calories per gram of protein) = Total number of protein grams recommended per day

UNDERSTANDING YOUR CARBOHYDRATES VALUES

Carbohydrates are known to be the body's "energy" providers and are critical in fueling our organs and central nervous system. There are many great carbohydrate choices available (with clean sources and low glycemic index levels); however, our modern-day society has made it too easy to provide us with carbohydrates that aren't always providing our diet with the best options. The RDA recommended dose for carbohydrates for females is a maximum of 130g per day with a recommended acceptable macronutrient distribution range (AMDR) of 45–65% a day.[20] With this AMDR recommendation range of 45–65%, it equates to a range of 225–325g of carbohydrates and a total of 900–1,300 calories.

Knowing that the protein requirement for a female would be somewhere around 30% (equating to around 600 calories per day at optimal levels), and without even considering the calories that will be coming from calculating the last macronutrient (fats), you can see how this average for carbohydrates is extremely high.

The ReShapeHER program suggests the carbohydrate recommendations at the lower end of the RDA's AMDR carbohydrate recommendation range of 40–45%. This allows a mother to consume the

recommended higher-end AMDR range for her protein consumption at 25-35%+, and still allows her enough calories for the day to include her healthy fats (the last macronutrient discussed below).

For the average female weighing 150 pounds and eating an average of 2,000 calories per day, this would equate to about 200–225 grams of carbohydrates per day, which would equate to a range of 800–900 total calories. The following calculation can be used to determine carbohydrate consumption:

Total calories per day x 40–45% = Total calories of carbohydrates recommended per day

Total calories of carbs recommended per day ÷ 4 (calories per gram of carbohydrate) = Total number of carbohydrate grams recommended per day

Oftentimes, females can consider carbohydrates and fats to be interchangeable in terms of how they disperse their calories after considering their protein requirements. Both of these macronutrients provide energy for the body; however, their energy values in terms of calorie contributions per gram differ dramatically. Fats contribute nine calories per gram versus carbohydrates at four calories per gram. Although they are both powerhouses in terms of how they supply the body energy, they do differ in terms of how they contribute to various bodily functions. It is important when considering these two macronutrients with the remainder of calories left in one's TDEE after their recommended protein consideration that they are also meeting the recommendations of carbohydrates and fats when doing so.

UNDERSTANDING YOUR FAT VALUES

Fats are the last macronutrient category and are critical, especially for women, in order to maintain hormonal health. Additionally, there are many benefits to "good" fats such as providing Omega-3 and Omega-6 that the human body is not able to create on its own and are important for cell membranes, and serving as precursors to many other substances in the body such as those involved in regulating blood pressure and inflammatory responses. These calories can easily add up if someone were to consume high levels of fat in their diet, which could result in a calorie surplus and also weight gain. Additionally, it is important to balance the amount of fats consumed so there is room for a balanced diet that also contains both of the other two types of macronutrients that are key to a healthy diet—protein and carbohydrates.

There is no recommended dietary allowance (RDA), adequate intake (AI), or total fat intake for any population other than infants. The acceptable macronutrient distribution range (AMDR) for fats is 20–35% for men and women ages 19 years and older (which would equate to 44–78 grams per day). Considering the above percentages for proteins and carbohydrates we used for our 150 pound female above, and also considering the RDA recommendations for fats, the ReShapeHER program leaves around 600 calories for a mother to stay within the higher end of the AMDR recommendations at 25-30% for fats (which equates to about 55-67 g per day).

The ReShapeHER program suggests a 25-30% overall calorie consumption to be fats for a female, equaling around 500-600 calories for the average 150-pound female.

The following formula can be used to calculate fats:

> Total calories per day x 25–30% = Total calories of fats recommended per day

Total calories of fats recommended per day ÷ 9 (calories per gram of fats) = Total fat grams recommended per day

Note: Alcohol is a non-nutrient that doesn't provide value in terms of macronutrients. However, for tracking purposes, its energy contribution (calories) can be tracked and benchmarked against your TDEE.

This can be done under fats (as its contribution in terms of kcals are closer to fats at 7kcal/g), by dividing the total calories of the drink by 9. Additionally, it can also be done under carbohydrates, by dividing the total calories of the drink by 4.

How the ReShapeHER Program Helps You Understand How to Calculate Your Macronutrients with one, simple CLICK!

Watch this video to find out how!

Note: these macronutrient values will fluctuate up and down as TDEE values do. Therefore, adjustments to TDEE will also reflect adjustments to macronutrient values.

As discussed in the video, once you have completed calculating your macronutrients values, these totals should equal your total TDEE (calories per day) when you sum them all up (based on grams). *The percentages you add up for each macronutrient should always equal 100% (which reflects that all three equal 100% of your TDEE value).* These values will be critical to enter into the tracking application you will use, in order to track your foods against these values. Regardless of whatever nutritional tracking system you use, you will always base your nutrition off your calculated values. The reason for this, is to allow you to be in control of your own values, as staying within these values will lead you to your nutritional goals.

Through successful nutritional tracking and experiencing how this results in changes with your body composition over time, you are able to understand why the lower end of the AMDR percentage recommendations for proteins can be challenged when it comes to our macronutrient consumption as a mother. Should a mother not consume enough protein, she will not be able to maintain and grow her muscles. Should she have a carbohydrate consumption that is too high, she won't have room for higher protein consumption and an ample amount of fats that support her hormones.

The ReShapeHER program suggests daily recommendations for each macronutrient for mothers: protein consumption at 25–35% of total daily calories, carbohydrate consumption at 40–45%, and a fat recommendation at 25–30%. Should a female choose to do so, she could raise or lower her carbohydrate intake by 5% (keeping her protein at a stable 30%) and still stay within her recommendations for fats. For example, should a woman decide she would like to set her protein intake at 30% and her carbohydrate intake at 45% in lieu of 40%, this would result in a fat intake of 25% overall total calories.

As I've stated before, our fitness is constantly in a fluid state. A mother's daily calories, and her macronutrient values that are included in this value, are the driver to her fitness goals. It is important to remember that when it comes to body fat loss or gain, daily calorie values determine what happens over time. However, it is also critical to remember that a mother's daily calories aren't representative of her entire fitness picture. It is still important to consume a balanced percentage of all three macronutrients as recommended in the ReShapeHER program, in order for her to support the functions her body needs to make, that will ultimately contribute to her fitness success.

There will be times that you will need to adjust these values, such as when your scale weight changes, you adjust your fitness goals, etc. These values are also highly individualized and can't be compared from one woman to another. This is because every woman's body is unique when it comes to her body composition and nutritional requirements. When you become more familiar with the process of knowing the values of the foods you're consuming, you will become an expert at knowing how your body responds to the balance of each macronutrient, and this in itself is an education that will serve you well in reaching your fitness goals over your lifetime. *Remember, a mother's TDEE values may change, also contributing to a change in all three of her macronutrient values, but her macronutrient percentages should not have to (unless a mother decides). A mother's total macronutrient percentages should always equal 100.*

THE IMPORTANCE OF NUTRITIONAL TRACKING

Becoming an expert in knowing your percentages and macronutrient distributions that result in your optimal fitness outcomes takes some time and patience. Also, as a mother's body changes, so do many other things like her requirements as well as her body composition responses to her macronutrient distributions. Practicing good nutrition, and understanding how to track this over time, not only gives us control of our bodies but also that of our overall health. It can be the greatest education we give ourselves as mothers when it comes to our overall fitness and possibly quality of life!

When it comes to nutritional tracking, it is important to understand that it's not just the quantity but also the QUALITY of what we are consuming that ultimately contributes to our overall health. Having a nutritional plan that consists of a good balance of all of the macronutrients that successfully fit within our required daily calories is key. Without a balance of quality macronutrients, this may result in a mother having a nutritional deficiency in her diet. A mother needs to remember that although weight loss may be warranted and attention needs to be paid to her daily calories in terms of a calorie deficit, an equal amount of attention should be paid to the QUALITY of macronutrients that make up her daily calories, in order for her to achieve her long-term fitness and health goals.

Patience is key when it comes to nutritional tracking. Just as every mother may differ in terms of her calorie and macronutrient requirements, they may also differ in terms of their individual responses to them and their adjustments. For example, a mother may put muscle on very quickly with an increase in her protein contribution to her diet, as well as with her fitness efforts, while another mother may do this much slower. We all have varying degrees of bodily responses to our dietary changes as our bodies adapt. Knowing how to give ourselves adequate time in order to evaluate our responses is key, which is why the ReShapeHER program recommends calorie adjustments every two to four weeks as weight changes.

It is also important to exercise patience with nutritional tracking, as it won't always give us precise values for what we're consuming. Even though we may do our best in terms of reading labels and basing our recipes and meals on exact portion sizing, there will always be room for error. Additionally, we won't always be in a situation that allows us to accurately track our food, such as restaurants, home gatherings, grabbing meals on the go, etc. However, through the practice of understanding how to track the foods we consume, we are more equipped to understand how to make better choices when it comes to our foods, and how much we are consuming which leads us to successful fitness outcomes.

When a mother doesn't have the education on how to successfully track her nutrition, she is just merely trying to shoot darts at a target in the dark when it comes to achieving her fitness goals. Considering our food consumption in general contributes around 80% to our overall daily calories (TDEE), you can see how critical it is for us to understand how to have a solid diet in order to reach our fitness goals. A mother could have a great fitness plan, but if it doesn't have a solid nutritional component based on tracking and understanding the values of the foods she's consuming, she will fail to have control in reaching her ultimate fitness goals. She may also put herself at risk for suffering from a variety of nutritional deficiencies that occur if she does not have enough of a particular macronutrient.

For example, without enough fats in her diet, this may wreak havoc on her hormones. (I know all of us mothers can appreciate balanced hormones!) Too little carbohydrates can leave a mother with "brain fog" and little energy. Most importantly, too little protein can ultimately result in a mother having muscle atrophy that later results in leaving her frail and suffering from diseases such as osteoporosis, etc. These health consequences and their importance when it comes to nutritional tracking far outweigh any weight loss attempts when it comes to the importance of why we should, as mothers, want to understand how to track our nutrition successfully.

Once a mother has gained the knowledge of how to track her nutrition successfully, she can then be a little more reliant on her intuition in terms of choosing foods that she knows will fulfill her personal dietary requirements based on her experience. She may at that point be able to better understand how to estimate portions and serving sizes. She may have a good idea about how she can base her satiety, fitness responses, etc. on the food choices she makes. However, in our modern-day society, our intuition when it comes to food is incredibly challenged. Marketing, advertising, our accessibility to food, our stressful environment, and many other things leave us with less time and more challenges in being successful with our intuition.

As busy mothers, we are often left to make impulse decisions when it comes to our food choices, as we tend to grab what is quick and easy. When it comes to food, we sometimes prioritize ourselves last to that of our family. Rather than being stuck in the muddied waters of our intuition derailing us from our fitness goals, nutritional tracking can serve as our beacon in the darkness of these challenges when it comes to our diet. We can simply get back on track and have control when our intuition fails us.

Whether we are tracking our nutrition or banking on our intuition, we have to remember that we can't outsmart a bad diet! Although diet and exercise contribute to fitness outcomes, a diet reigns far supreme and calories will always win. However, it is critical for us to always remember that fitness, and overall health outcomes, are reliant on the quality of these calories. The quality of wholesome foods that we eat will fuel our fitness efforts. More often than not, our calorie contributions or deficits that we make in terms of our fitness are largely made with diet more than our movement. Our general idea of how much we contribute to our fitness in terms of our movements (planned movements specifically—EAT) are generally grossly overrated when compared to the contributions our diets can make in terms of our overall calorie outputs. This is the reason why you may know a fellow mother who is generally very active and works out but struggles when it comes to weight loss.

In my opinion, nutritional tracking can counteract the bad relationships that can often be established with mothers and food. It is a practice that can allow a mother to enjoy any type of food as it fits within her nutritional requirements, versus avoiding certain foods that may have been demonized in the past or labeled as "bad foods" she felt she couldn't enjoy. I know from personal experience with my own mother suffering from her bad relationship with food how damaging these food labels can be and how it can lead to feelings of shame and guilt. I often wonder how different things would have been growing up had my mother had an education about nutritional tracking and how this could have enabled her to control her fitness outcomes.

Tracking your calories and macronutrients won't guarantee that you'll live a life of zero health issues, but what it does allow you is an opportunity to understand the critical nutrients (and in what amounts) your body needs in order to support your best health outcomes. According to the National Institute of Health in their *PubMed* article on dietary tracking, "dietary tracking was found to be an important component of successful weight loss, with those who tracked at least 5 days of each week showing significant and sustained weight loss over time as compared to those who tracked fewer days or inconsistently during the program. Consistent tracking is a significant predictor of weight loss, resulting in additional seven pounds of weight loss over the course of the program suggesting the intervention successfully achieved clinically and significant long-term weight loss in high-risk rural Appalachian adults with diabetes and prediabetes."[21]

SUMMARY

Congratulations! You are now in the driver's seat of your fitness goals by taking the time to read and understand the information in this chapter! Through your knowledge, you can appreciate how nutritional tracking can help you realize how your overall nutrition contributes to your fitness outcomes. You are now aware that by being patient, disciplined, and honest with yourself, you will see results through this practice. Through the process of nutritional tracking, you can confidently combat the pitfall of having a poor diet because you won't be blindly making efforts toward your nutrition, contributing to the pitfall of "The Poor Diet" you read about in this chapter. You now understand how the ReShapeHER program, and the education it provides a mother through this practice, that any mother can successfully achieve her nutrition and fitness goals in a short period of time.

CHAPTER 6 CLIFF NOTES

- Calculating your Total Daily Energy Expenditure (TDEE) will help you understand the calories (in terms of energy) your body needs to maintain itself. A lower TDEE per day (fewer calories consumed through diet or fewer calories as a result of higher calorie outputs contributed through exercise/movements) results in body weight/fat loss. A higher TDEE (more calories consumed through diet or more calories as a result of less calorie outputs contributed through exercise/movements) results in body weight/fat gain.
- Our total daily energy expenditure (TDEE), which we often think of in terms of the daily calories our body burns, determines how much of all three macronutrients we can consume.
- Although energy balance (your TDEE) reigns supreme no matter what you eat, you will gain with a calorie surplus and lose with a calorie deficit.
- Knowing how to successfully calculate and balance all three macronutrients (protein, carbohydrates and fats), allows us to consume proper amounts that support our necessary bodily functions, promoting good health and leading us to achieve the body composition we desire.
- Each macronutrient plays a specific role in bodily functions and each one is important to consume in healthy amounts as determined by our TDEE.
- Their thermogenic effects, their ability to contribute the most to muscle maintenance and growth, as well as to increase a mother's satiety, is why the ReShapeHER program prioritizes proteins first when it comes to nutritional tracking.
- When calculating the healthy consumption of macronutrients,

it is important to consider their energy contributions (Proteins—4kcal/g, Carbohydrates—4kcal/g, Fats—9kcal/g).

- The ReShapeHER program sets solid daily recommendations for protein consumption at 25-35%, carbohydrate consumption at 40-45% and a fat recommendation at 25-30% of total daily calories (all within AMDR percentage recommendations for women).
- A mother's TDEE values may change, also contributing to a change in all three of her macronutrient values, but her macronutrient percentages within these values do not have to. A mother's total macronutrient percentages should always equal 100%.
- It is important to understand that our fitness is in a fluid state! Adjustments to both our TDEE and macronutrient values will need to be made over time, with things such as scale weight changes, changing fitness goals, etc. These values are also highly individualized and can't be compared from one woman to another!.
- Nutritional tracking helps us understand to the greatest capacity how our nutrition contributes to our fitness outcomes.
- The ReShapeHER program makes it easy for a mother to obtain and understand her TDEE values in one, simple CLICK! (*watch video to find out how*!)
- The ReShapeHER program makes it easy for a mother to obtain and understand her Macronutrient values in one, simple CLICK! (*watch video to find out how!*)

NOTES

NOTES

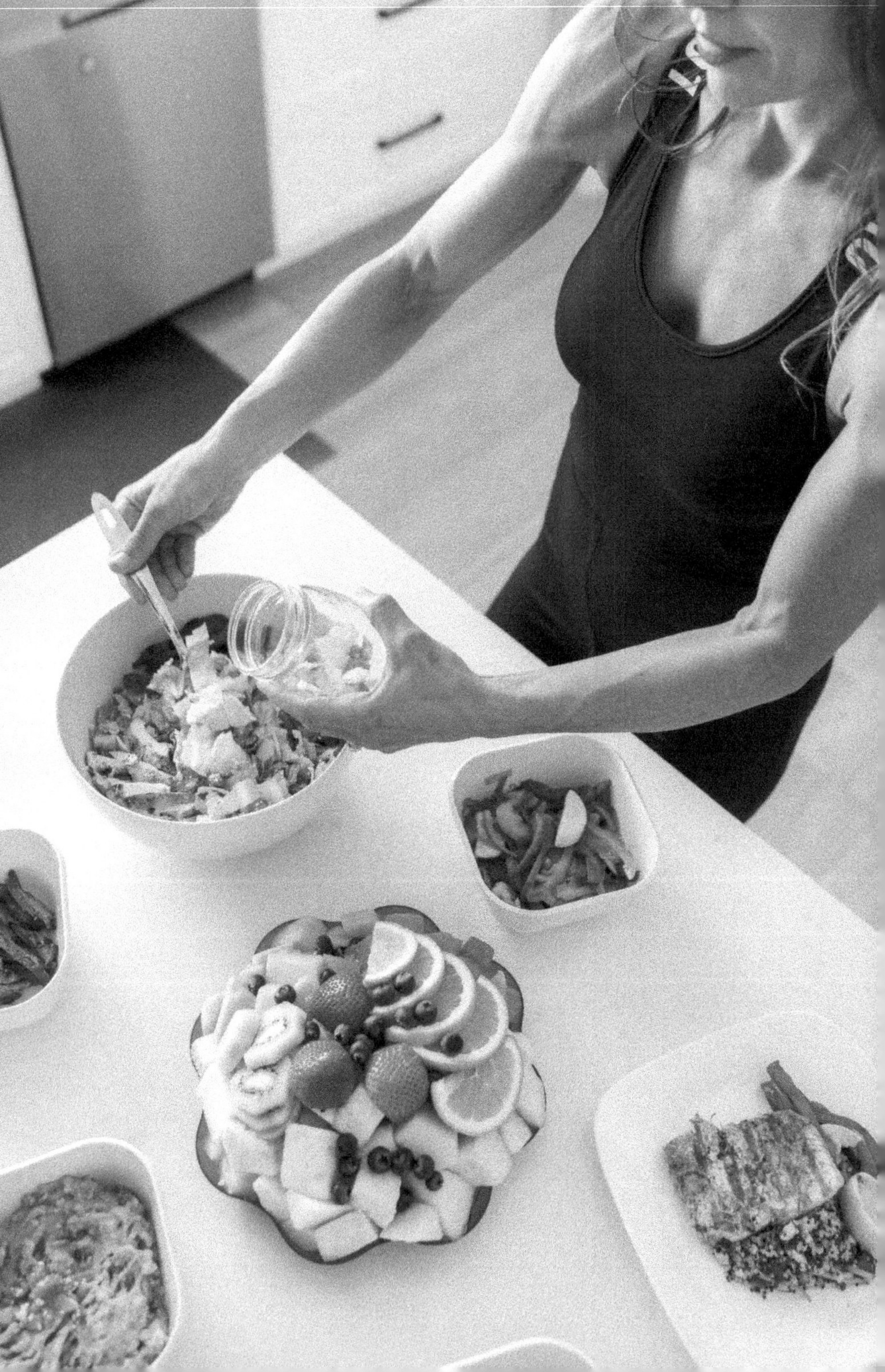

7

Combating Pitfall #2

—The Yo-Yo Diet

IN THIS CHAPTER, I DISCUSS another common pitfall mothers fall prey to. . . "The Yo-Yo Diet". It is often turned to because of the lack of education that I discussed in the previous chapter. This diet is commonly practiced, not only because of a lack of fitness education, but also due to our lack of patience and being fixated on instantaneous results. Unfortunately, it is not a sustainable practice, and although it can be temporarily successful, it puts us at risk when it comes to the detriments it places on our long-term health.

As mothers, if we understand how we can effectively control our fitness outcomes, allowing us to make healthy and manageable changes over time, we can avoid this common pitfall. With the education in the ReShapeHER program, a mother is able to have the confidence in knowing how she can control her nutritional values to reach her overall fitness goals. This chapter discusses the third and final value that will allow her to do this, through understanding and calculating her daily caloric intake based on her **Season**.

In this chapter, I discuss the basic principles of how a mother will choose a **Season** based on her fitness goals through the practice of nutritional tracking. I discuss how a mother can do these calculations on her own, or simply click the video at the end of this chapter, to easily apply the information she's learned in this chapter.

A SEASONAL APPROACH TO NUTRITION

In this chapter, I will discuss one of the ways a mother can tailor her nutritional needs to her goals through a seasonal approach to her diet and fitness. These seasons are best thought of like the weather. We usually experience all of them and our clothing and practices change and adjust, just as they do. The same can be said with fitness seasons... they each have their own purpose and they repeat over and over again, as goals are reached. With the ReShapeHER program, a mother can decide what season she is in with her fitness journey, based on her goals. Regardless of this season, the ReShapeHER program will provide her a guide, right at her fingertips, all based on her individualized information. As her goals change, she can simply adjust her season as this program provides her all of the information she will need to successfully accomplish this.

The ultimate goal of having seasons is to achieve one's best body composition. Body composition is our state of "tone," which is a state of our bodies being constantly in "flux" and results in a healthy balance of body fat and muscle tissue. By working on this balance with our efforts of reducing or maintaining our body fat and/or maintaining or growing our muscle, we develop a better body composition over time. Each season differs in terms of its contribution and goals as they relate to our total daily energy expenditure (TDEE) when it comes to diet, as well as with our movements and planned exercise. For example, the TDEE goal in an "on" season (sometimes called "prep" season, "dieting" season, etc.) is to create a conservative calorie deficit over time, in order to drive fat loss. The TDEE goal in an "off" season (sometimes called "bulking" season, although this name may have contributed to mothers avoiding it) is to create a conservative calorie surplus over time, in order to drive lean muscle gain and keep body fat gain at a minimum. The TDEE goal in a "maintenance" season, is to remain at status quo with calories, in order to support one's current body composition. Below I will discuss how the ReShapeHER program sets a mother's TDEE goals based on her season.

Along with calories, the exercise part of a fitness plan differs with each season. A mother in an "on" season may choose to do more cardiovascular or NEAT movements (discussed later in this book) to drive the calorie deficit she is trying to make. Conversely, she may choose not to do as much movement in her "off" season to support the muscle growth, having it result mainly from her resistance training in lieu of cardiovascular activities. The ReShapeHER program includes a fitness outline that can be tailored to any mother's season and busy lifestyle, through the 3-Day and 5-Day Fitness Plans (discussed in a later chapter). Through resistance training, cardiovascular and NEAT exercises recommendations, a mother can contribute more or less of her time to these depending on the fitness season she is in.

I discuss how a mother can accomplish her seasonal calculations on her own below. Otherwise, she can simply click on the video at the end of this section to find out how she can SIMPLY obtain her seasonal daily caloric intake (TDEE) with the ReShapeHER program!

HOW TO SET YOUR TOTAL DAILY ENERGY EXPENDITURE (TDEE) TO YOUR SEASON WITH THE RESHAPEHER PROGRAM

1 | "On" Season – Fat Loss/Muscle Maintenance

In this season, your primary goal is fat loss. Your focus isn't on growing your lean muscle tissue as much as it is on reducing your overall body fat. You will be focused solely on maintaining a CALORIE DEFICIT (reduction of calories from your TDEE, which also lowers your macronutrient values). Although you can still grow muscle tissue in this season, it is not done as effectively as in an "off" season (calorie surplus) or "maintenance" season (calories remain at or around TDEE). Your goal isn't to remain in this season for a long period of time, as your body would start the process of metabolic adaptation, that would work against your fitness goals. Your ultimate priority in this season is to have a specific fat loss goal, execute fitness and nutritional goals based on this goal, and quickly return back to your "maintenance" season once your goal has been accomplished in order to avoid adaptation. Because of this, the ReShapeHER program recommends a conservative deficit of 10–20% reduction in overall TDEE calories, (which should equate to about 0.5—1 pound weight loss per week). *This TDEE value needs to be recalculated and possibly adjusted every 2–4 weeks due to possible weight and body composition changes.* Also, because your body is always in flux, don't assume that your TDEE will be the same from one "on" season to the next!

How to Calculate for your "On" Season:

(You will use your TDEE value from Chapter 4)

TDEE x 0.1 or 0.2 = Deficit Value (reflecting a 10% or 20% reduction in calories)

TDEE – Deficit Value = Total "on" season TDEE

A mother's TDEE must be recalculated and possibly adjusted every 2-4 weeks (critical due to weight changes)

"Diet Breaks" recommended for 1-2 days, every 3-4 weeks

2 | "Off" Season – Muscle Growth

In this season, your primary goal is muscle growth. You may be entering this season because you've been dieting down too long and have lost muscle or just to gain more muscle overall, to contribute to your overall tone. Your focus isn't on losing body fat (as you WILL NOT LOSE WEIGHT IN A CALORIE SURPLUS) but rather growing lean muscle tissue to allow for better tone after you exit this stage and go into an "on" season in order to lean out. You will be focused on being in a conservative calorie surplus in order to support the energy demands your body will need to do the exercises (specifically resistance training) that will support this muscle growth. The ReShapeHER program recommends a conservative 10–15% increase above a mother's TDEE in order for her to develop lean muscle tissue but also avoid gaining unnecessary body fat, (this should equate to about 0.5—1 pound per week). *This TDEE value needs to be recalculated and possibly adjusted every 2-4 weeks due to possible weight and body composition changes.* Also, because your body is always in flux, don't assume that your TDEE will be the same from one "off" season to the next!

How to Calculate your TDEE for an "Off" Season:

TDEE x 0.1 or 0.2 = Surplus Value (reflecting a 10% or 20% increase in calories)

TDEE + Surplus Value = Total "Off" season TDEE

A mother's TDEE must be recalculated and possibly adjusted every 2-4 weeks (critical due to weight changes)

3 | "Maintenance" Season – Status Quo

- Serves as your "status quo" when reaching idealistic body composition after a successful "on" season or "off" season.
- Can be used as a "diet break" (suggested 1-2 days every 2-4 weeks) while in a calorie deficit ("on" season) or calorie surplus ("off" season).
- Serves as your long-term goal once you've achieved your ideal body composition!

In this season, your primary goal is to maintain the status quo (same weight and body composition) in terms of your body composition. It is important to remember that after an "on" or "off" season, your "maintenance" weight will be the ending weight for these seasons. This new weight will most likely be different with either of these two seasons, so this is important to note, as this new weight will determine your new "maintenance" season baseline. Keeping calories at maintenance will not support body fat loss; however, they can still support conservative muscle growth (although not as effectively as a calorie surplus in an "off" season). However, should you decide to not do resistance training yet keep calories at status quo, muscle tissue will be lost, which is why it's critical to continue to do resistance training! Additionally, should your diet not consist of quality macronutrients even though you have the same calorie intake, your body composition will also suffer as you won't be eating the right nutrients to support muscle and aid in a healthy body fat percentage. However, when done correctly, this season is also your ultimate goal when achieving your ideal body composition by going through the other two seasons. *However, considering your body is always in flux and our nutritional and fitness tracking is not always precise, it is important to recalculate and possibly adjust a maintenance TDEE over time (this depends on the individual and their circumstances).* Also, because your body is always in flux, don't assume that your TDEE will be the same from one "maintenance" season to the next!

How to Calculate your TDEE for a "Maintenance" Season:

TDEE = YOUR DAILY CALCULATED TDEE (SEE CHAPTER 6) *May need to be recalculated over time with weight fluctuations*

How the ReShapeHER Program Helps You Understand How to Calculate Your TDEE for your Season with one, simple CLICK!

Watch this video to find out how!

bitly

Note: these macronutrient values will fluctuate up and down as TDEE values do. Therefore, adjustments to TDEE will also reflect adjustments to macronutrient values.

SOME BULLET POINTS ON SEASONS:

- A mother can still achieve muscle growth in her "maintenance" season (she DOES NOT have to be in an "off" season/calorie surplus to accomplish this). It is a more slower process for a mother to grow muscle in a maintenance season (especially if she isn't a beginner).
- A mother's overall movement enables her to create a calorie deficit with respect to her TDEE and less movement could create a calorie surplus (if she consumes over what her movement creates in terms of a calorie output).
- Weight loss is not just driven by a mother's movement, but also by the number of calories she consumes. By consuming less calories than her TDEE (irrespective of her movement), she will lose weight. By consuming more calories than her TDEE over time, she will gain weight.
- A mother can use **BOTH** her movement and calories consumed, to drive overall weight loss.
- Although the ReShapeHER program is effective in helping a mother understand her overall TDEE requirements based on her lifestyle and fitness goals, there is still room for error. It is critical for a mother to understand her own calculations and individual requirements as she progresses in her fitness journey in order to reach her goals. This can only be effectively done with time and consistency.
- In order to determine true fitness progress in terms of weight loss, it's critical for a mother to understand her body composition values to ensure that this weight loss isn't being driven by muscle loss but rather fat loss.

FITNESS SEASONS—PUTTING IT ALL TOGETHER

I've discussed how your body composition is always fluid in previous chapters. As your body changes (in terms of your scale weight), your TDEE will need to be recalculated and possibly adjusted. For example, if you calculated your TDEE and macronutrients based on the weight you are today and lost some weight over time, both your TDEE and macronutrient values would need to be possibly lowered, as your "maintenance" weight would have changed. The reason for this, is that at a lower body weight, fewer calories are required for it to function (therefore your TDEE and macronutrient requirements would be lower). Conversely, if you gained muscle and also weight, your TDEE calorie requirements could be higher. This is why the ReShapeHER program recommends a mother recalculates and possibly adjusts her TDEE to her goals, every two to four weeks.

It is also important to note that if your activity level has changed regardless of the season you're in, this will also affect your TDEE as you are contributing more toward your calorie input or output (this is calculated by adjusting your activity multiplier). If you are less active, you would need to lower your TDEE requirements. In contrast, higher activity would allow you to raise your TDEE requirements in order to stay at your desired weight.

At any point during a "calorie surplus" or "calorie deficit" phase, a woman can determine her new "maintenance" TDEE to support her current weight and simply adjust her TDEE and macronutrient values to reflect what that is, if she desires to remain there. However, over time, should her weight move up or down from this established "maintenance" weight, her TDEE (and also her macronutrients values within this number) would then need to be adjusted again based on her fitness goals. For example, if a 150-pound female has a TDEE of let's say 2,000 calories, if she loses five pounds, her TDEE will also adjust and be less, because she has less weight that has to be supported with her energy requirements. Conversely, should this 150-pound female choose to be in an "off" season and gain five pounds, she would need a slightly greater surplus to support the energy demands for her higher weight. This is the reason why losing weight, and keeping it off, can be especially challenging for mothers and females in general. It is always critical to respect our bodies as mothers, knowing that our fitness is always in a fluid state that needs continual adjusting over time.

There are many factors that may affect a female's scale weight that aren't so crystal clear (such as inflammation, hormonal fluctuations, menstruation, stress levels, the aging process, etc.) that may require us to make adjustments to our TDEE and macronutrient values, which we may have less control of. These are many of the reasons why the ReShapeHER supports conservative adjustments in one's TDEE and macronutrient values, as this allows the body to make appropriate changes over time successfully. These factors that affect women regularly can cause stress on their bodies. Should we compound this stress with an aggressive calorie surplus or deficit, we could exponentially add to a woman's stress load and derail her from meeting her fitness goals. It is critical to remember the phenomena that I've discussed in the previous chapter about metabolic adaptation. The body is incredibly effective at trying to find a balance and adapting to the conditions it is put under. Should a woman try to aggressively practice a calorie surplus or deficit, it renders the body to defend itself and quickly find ways to adapt, derailing a woman from reaching her fitness goals. Patience and a conservative approach is key!

It is important for a Mother to keep in mind what each season serves to accomplish, and what her expectations should be with each one. When a mother is in "off" season (calorie surplus), a natural amount of body fat will accompany lean muscle tissue gain. This is a normal and expected occurrence. Because developing lean muscle tissue is her goal, she will embrace this occurrence, knowing that after a successful "off" season, she will follow this with an "on" season to lose the body fat that was gained in order for her to achieve a better body composition. She will know that it will be critical to embrace her body regardless of the conservative addition of body fat, knowing that with the ReShapeHER program, will be making successful efforts in sculpting the body composition she wants to achieve.

During an "on" season (calorie deficit), a mother's body will oftentimes fight against her efforts in losing body fat as it transitions into a new season. She might not often see results in terms of weight loss, as it works hard to conserve calories knowing it's in a conservative deficit. She may sometimes feel hungrier while it adjusts and with a lesser amount of calories and not as energetic as she was in an "off" season. She may need to consider more unplanned exercise (NEAT) in this area, as it may require lesser amounts of our energy than our planned exercise (EAT) and has a greater contribution toward her calorie expenditure (a whopping 15% versus 5%!). A mother in this season, despite her energy levels, will need to continue her resistance training so she can maintain her lean muscle tissue while losing body fat. She will have to spend additional time nutritional tracking more precisely and eating the correct foods that fuels her fitness efforts, knowing her TDEE is lower than it once was. All of these things should be expected and also the reason why this season shouldn't last a mother a long time, knowing that with the ReShapeHER program and through her consistent efforts, she will reach her fitness goals.

In "maintenance" season, a mother will understand how critical it will be to stay within her personal TDEE to maintain her current body composition through your ongoing nutrition and fitness efforts. She will learn to appreciate that "maintenance" season is her ultimate goal, knowing that she is satisfied with her body composition and understands exactly how to support it with the ReShapeHER program.

When it comes to fitness seasons, a mother can easily change them with the ReShapeHER program, along with your fitness goals. For example, should she lose body fat and realize that she'd like to have better muscle tone, she can switch from "on" season to "off" season by adjusting her fitness and dietary requirements based on her TDEE. Conversely, should she feel like she's made enough contributions toward a healthy amount of lean muscle tissue, she can switch from "off" season to "on" season in order to conservatively lose body fat and achieve the body composition she desires. Lastly, she can always choose to stay in "maintenance" season at any point, to simply maintain her current body composition and even slowly make advancements towards her muscle growth. The ReShapeHER program gives a mother the outline to tailor her season to whatever goal she'd like to achieve.

IMPORTANT SECRETS TO KNOW ABOUT SEASONS

Knowing How to Let Metabolic Adaptation Work in Your Favor—Your Calorie "Ceiling"

The ReShapeHER program understands the science of metabolic adaptation and incorporates this into the plan so mothers can achieve success. One of the greatest ways mothers can have success is by understanding how to have a great "off" season and build up their calorie "ceiling". What this means is that by following the ReShapeHER conservative "off" season recommendations, they can successfully drive up the amount of calories they are able to consume for their individual body weight over time. With a conservative approach, this allows a mother to consume more calories over time for her body weight, without gaining unnecessary body fat. As a mother puts on more muscle, she is able to improve her metabolism and possibly burn more calories for her body weight, allowing her to possibly increase her TDEE. A mother obtains a higher TDEE in "off" season by successfully optimizing resistance training for her lean muscle tissue development, as well as having an optimal macronutrient distribution which supports her healthy body fat percentage. She will continue to take conservative calorie surpluses over time (recalculating and possibly adjusting their TDEE every 2-4 weeks) and understanding her body composition values, to ensure she is meeting her goals. Finally, when she has completed this type of "off" season successfully, she will be able to enter an "on" season with a much higher TDEE than she had previously, which allows her to have an easier time dieting down as she enjoys a higher amount of calories during her "on" season.

Personally, when I was able to drive up my calories to about 3,000 daily in my "off" season, I ended with my lowest calories per day being only 1,850 in my following "on" season and was able to Nationally qualify in Bodybuilding. I used the art of science to almost reverse the metabolic adaptation my body would have succumbed to had I ended my "on" season at a lower TDEE or practiced it too aggressively in general. This is the reason why successful female bodybuilders are able to compete year after year. They understand that with a conservative approach and the understanding of how to program their fitness and diet programs, they can endure the many seasons it takes for them to reach their goals. This is also the reason why these bodybuilders don't discuss their TDEE requirements, as they know how individualized they are and how they can't be compared depending on one's approach and experience. The ReShapeHER program incorporates these concepts and tailors them to a mother so that she can reap the same benefits as these successful female bodybuilders!

The Art of "Diet Breaks"

Lastly, one of the secrets the ReShapeHER program includes is how to use the "maintenance" season to a mother's advantage. The art of doing "diet breaks" (a short period of time in which someone will consume calories at their maintenance TDEE in order to avoid metabolic adaptation during a dieting phase or "on" season), is key when combating the metabolic adaptation that can take place when dieting. Taking a diet break can trick the body into thinking it's not in a calorie deficit by allowing for more energy to support its efforts during dieting and the metabolic stress that it creates with a continual calorie deficit.

Additionally, these breaks can also be used to combat the stress of an "on" or "off" season. For example, should someone experience fatigue or exhaustion during "on" season, they can take a day or two in "maintenance" season to bring their calories back up, allowing for the extra energy to decrease the fatigue and aid in the exhaustion they may be experiencing in their workouts.

Taking diet breaks requires patience, as when they are included, they require more time for a mother to reach her body composition goals when it comes to fat loss. However, they are powerful tools when it comes to the long-term, as they allow mothers to reap the benefits of entering an "on" season with higher calories, not forcing her to drive her TDEE really low while dieting. The ReShapeHER program suggests that a diet break is incorporated during on-season 1-2 days every 3-4 weeks in order to avoid this adaptation.

CHAPTER 7 CLIFF NOTES

- One of the greatest ways a mother can tailor her nutritional needs to her goals is through a "seasonal" approach to her diet and fitness.
- Each season differs in terms of its contribution and goals as they relate to a mother's total daily energy expenditure (TDEE) when it comes to diet, as well as with our planned exercise and movements. The TDEE goal in "on" season is to create a conservative calorie deficit over time, in order to drive fat loss. The TDEE goal in "off" season is to create a conservative calorie surplus over time, in order to drive muscle gain and keep body fat gain at a minimum. The TDEE goal in "maintenance" season, is to keep calories at status quo, to support a mother's current physique.
- The ReShapeHER program makes it easy for a mother to understand her "seasonal" TDEE with one, simple CLICK!
- It is important to understand that recalculations with possible adjustments to a mother's total daily energy expenditure (TDEE), is not only done once but many times throughout her fitness journey as body composition and goals change! As weight fluctuates, so do our TDEE requirements.
- Both diet and exercise directly affect our TDEE in terms of calorie inputs and outputs.
- Our unplanned exercise (NEAT), often requires a lesser amount of energy than our planned exercise (EAT) and has a greater contribution towards our calorie expenditure (a whopping 15% versus 5%!)
- It is important for a mother to keep in mind what each season serves to accomplish, and what her expectations should be with

each one. She can switch from "on" season to "off" season by adjusting her fitness and dietary requirements based on her TDEE.

- A mother can make even greater contributions towards her fitness goals by understanding how to let metabolic adaptation work in her favor with her "off" season and also by understanding how to incorporate "diet breaks" into her "on" season.
- A solid nutritional plan, like the one in the ReShapeHER program, helps a mother avoid the yo-yo dieting pitfalls, allowing her to control her nutritional choices with confidence as she works towards obtaining her fitness goals.

NOTES

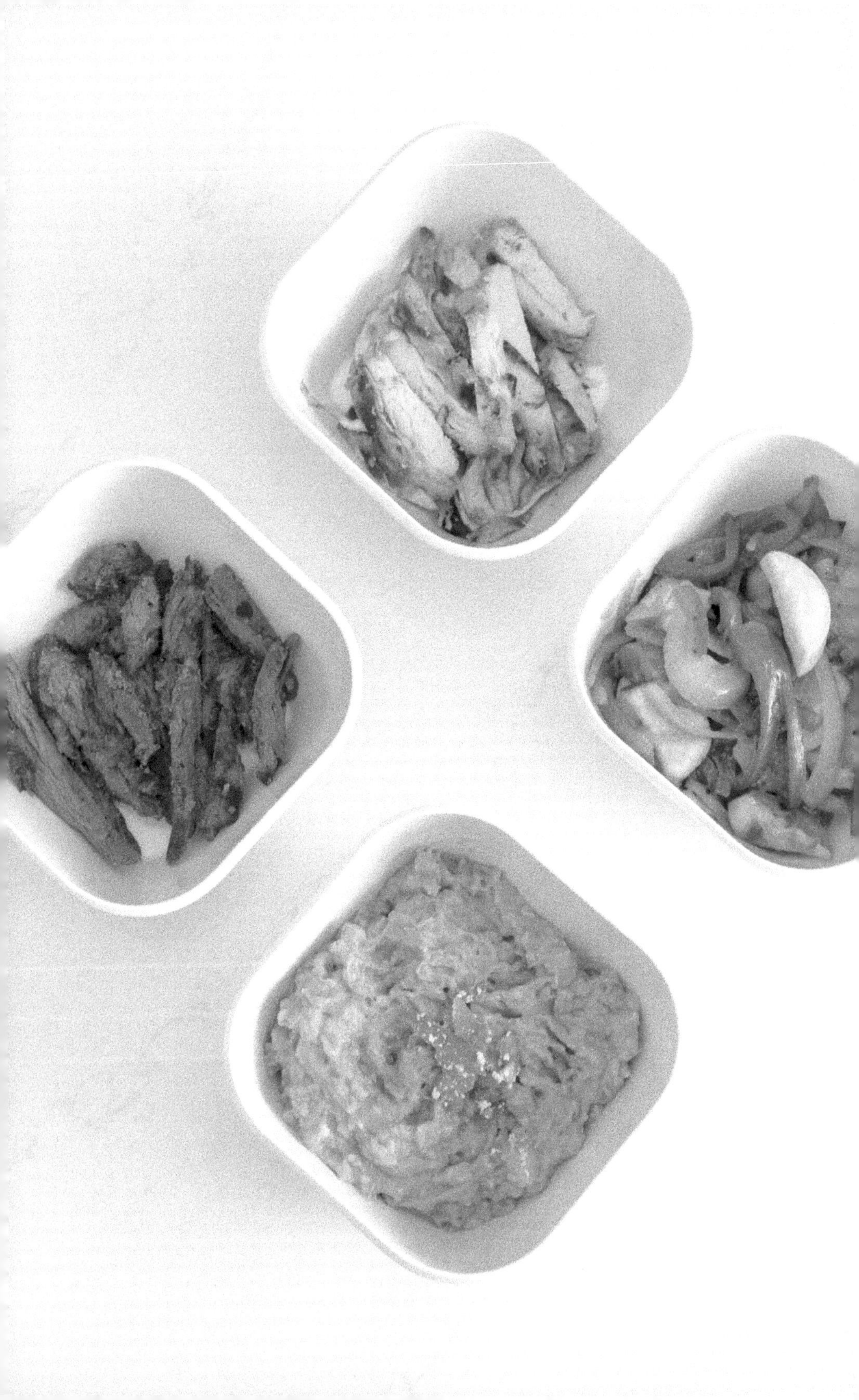

8

Nutritional Tracking Tools and Tips

YOU MIGHT BE THINKING BY this point... "I have all of my individualized nutritional values to reach my goals, but now what?" This chapter will break it all down for you, to understand how these numbers result in what ends up on your plate. However, it is critical to remember that this process is not a precise one. No matter how hard we may try as mothers, we will end up consuming more or less of the things we didn't intend. This is life. The goal isn't to be perfect, but rather make the majority of our efforts in the right direction in order to meet our goals. The important thing to note is that with the ReShapeHER program, you are being supported with knowing what these values need to be in terms of your nutrition and how you will use these values to achieve the body composition you desire in a short time!

There are many nutritional trackers available that allow you to enter your TDEE and macronutrient goals based on your body composition, (this was demonstrated in the ReShapeHER calculation videos). These nutritional trackers are great tools in that they allow for you to input the foods that you are consuming on a daily basis in order to understand how they are contributing toward your TDEE and macronutrient goals. (I will continue to use the MyFitnessPal app example throughout this book, as this is the one in which I am most familiar),[22] Regardless of the nutritional tracker you use, the important thing is that no matter which one, you are keeping track of your TDEE and macronutrient values on a daily basis to ensure that your efforts result in the health and body composition goals that you desire!

MYFITNESSPAL FUNCTIONALITIES

There are many areas of this application that you can use, to support your nutrition and fitness goals. I will mention the ones below, that are the most critical to understand when it comes to the ReShape-HER program:

DIARY SECTION:

1. Daily food items can be entered in one of three ways in your DIARY section in the MyFitnessPal app.

    a. By scanning their barcodes (the easiest and most accurate way).

    b. They can be searched in the system. By doing this, you will go under your Breakfast, Lunch, Dinner or snack section and click "add food." *Note: it's critical to make sure that your food searched and entered, is reflective of your correct serving size, same food brand or restaurant meal and matches any known nutritional value you many have on the particular food/meal. Remember, with any application like this, there is always room for human error!*

    c. They can be entered by recipe (each ingredient entered individually and then saved under "My Meals" or "My Recipes"). *Once you've spent the time entering the foods you often eat, the process of searching them up and inputting them into your diary section becomes much quicker and easier!*

2. Your DIARY section also provides you a tab on the bottom to enter your food and exercise notes for the day. You can use this to track your food notes (not to take the place of logging your

foods) as well as exercise notes (your workout for the day, etc.) You could even connect a step tracker under the "Exercise" section of this page!

3. The nutrition tab on the bottom of the diary page, will give you the ability to see your Daily or Weekly breakdown, in terms of your overall calories, nutrients and macros (you can even access and export your Complete Diary from the bottom of this page!)

GOALS SECTION:

1. You will enter your current and goal weight under your goals section. *It is critical to remember what you've learned in this book regarding scale weight. It doesn't reflect our body composition, so we need to consider this when choosing an arbitrary number!*

2. A weekly goal will be chosen in this section, in terms of how much weight loss (or gain) is desired per week. *The ReShapeHER program supports a weight loss/gain goal of 0.5–1 lb per week only.*

3. An activity level will be chosen in this section to reflect a mother's calorie expenditure (calories burned). This will be benchmarked against a mother's consumption (foods entered). *The ReShapeHER program's 3-Day and 5-Day fitness plans, would put a mother in the "active" fitness category for this section. It is critical to remember that if this activity level changes, her goals would need to be adjusted.*

4. Under the "Nutritional Goals" section, a mother can simply click the first section, that takes her to her overall calorie and macronutrient goals. Her calories will already be set based on what she entered for her goal weight and activity level. However, it's here that she can adjust her macronutrient percentages. She can simply click on each macronutrient percentage, and manually enter what she'd like them to be. *The ReShapeHER Program supports a macronutrient percentage for proteins to be 25-35%, carbohydrates to be 40-45% and fats to be 25-30% per day.* Once a mother returns

to her diary section, she will see that this information will be populated for her at the top of the page.

PROGRESS SECTION:

1. Scale weight readings can be entered under this section, by clicking the plus button at the top of the page. It is here that a mother can enter her weight, the date and also be able to attach a progress photo.

2. Scale weights are plotted in graph form, over the course of a week to over one year (you can change these time increments according to what you want to see). Additionally, these entries are populated on the bottom so you can revisit them and photos or reports can be exported.

MyFitnessPal offers many other functionalities in their application that I won't spend time discussing in this book, including ideas for recipes, meal planning and access to a community of fitness enthusiasts. It's a great application to track your nutrition and fitness, and one that has worked well for me in reaching my fitness goals successfully.

Author disclaimer: Since the publication of this book, I have no association with MyFitnessPal other than using it for my own personal fitness tracking.

Daily Calorie and Macronutrient Adjustments

When it comes to your daily calories (TDEE), remember that this number will need to be recalculated and possibly adjusted every 2-4 weeks as weight goes up and down. This will therefore change the values (in terms of grams) of the macronutrient allotments. As you move along in your season, you may also choose to change the percentage contributions of the macronutrients based on your fitness goals. For example, you may want to make a greater contribution toward your lean muscle tissue, so your protein and carbohydrate contribution of 25% and 45% may change to 30% and 40%. You can make these types of adjustments to any of the three macronutrients, as long as they all total a 100% contribution. Regardless of the adjustments you make, I always encourage conservative ones, so that you can more accurately understand how these adjustments are contributing to your body composition over time. If enough time isn't allowed, you won't be able to answer this question. Since I am mostly familiar with the MyFitnessPal app, I know it allows for a minimum of a 5% addition or reduction to each macronutrient.[23]

Plating and Percentages

Once you begin tracking your macronutrients, you'll start to understand how much of each macronutrient you'll need to achieve your goal from not only a plating perspective but also that of a volume one. You'll start to see your macronutrient percentage contributions play out in your daily eating habits, as your meals will start looking like their percentages. For example, with my personal 40/30/30 percent contributions of carbs/proteins/fats, most of my meals have a lean protein, complex carbohydrate, and healthy fat. Examples of my favorite meals include: grilled chicken with rice and vegetables, turkey meatballs with marinara sauce and gluten-free pasta, steak tacos with avocado, salsa, and polenta, etc.

Some of your meals may fall outside of your ideal macronutrient percentages, and this is fine! What you'll learn to do throughout each day is how to drive each macronutrient percentage closer to what it needs to be, by educating yourself on your food choices that contribute to them. For example, I love to have a larger carbohydrate meal in the morning (I like to do this, as the carbohydrates fuel my workouts that I typically do right after breakfast). My breakfast is often oatmeal with powdered peanut butter or granola of some sort with half of a protein bar. Because my first meal is higher in carbs, I make sure my lunch has fewer carbs and more protein. For example, my lunches tend to be salads with chicken (with no croutons or bread), lunch meats (minus the bread), with cottage cheese or yogurt, etc. As I've discussed in the previous chapter, nutritional tracking gives you the control to understand how to reach your fitness goals regardless of whatever season you are in.

Food Choices Based on Seasons

As you continue to grow in your knowledge about how to track your nutrition, you will start to understand how you can adjust this practice to your fitness season. This practice will allow you to successfully plan your meals according to your fitness goals. You won't have to play the guessing game when it comes to trying to achieve your fitness goals with your food choices.

Ultimately, this knowledge allows you to be in the driver seat when it comes to knowing how to control your food choices, regardless of what your lifestyle may be.

You will begin to understand and appreciate that with a conservative "off" season, you can enjoy a time in which you can be more liberal with your food choices as consume slightly more calories per day, making sure you are still making good food choices and macronutrient contributions towards your diet to ensure you are making proper muscle growth. Should you go beyond your daily TDEE, you will understand that your weight will increase as it gains a conservative amount of body fat gained in addition to muscle tissue with adequate protein consumption and resistance training. You will understand that if you don't meet your TDEE over time (especially in terms of your protein), you may not make the gains you were hoping to achieve. With additional calories, you will appreciate that meeting your protein requirements becomes easier. You'll learn that lean meats and other protein sources are great choices during "off" season as they are in your "on" season, and carbohydrates and fats continue to be essential in fueling your workouts and providing you with an ample amount of energy. By consistently tracking, you will be able to make better food choices over time through your knowledge and enjoy everything this season has to offer.

Through nutritional tracking, you will understand that although "on" season is the season that can be very challenging at times (depending on how far along you are and/or what type of calorie deficit you are in), you can achieve a successful one. There will be fewer calories to work with on a daily basis, but you'll know how to make the most impact towards your fitness goals with what you're allotted. You'll learn to appreciate nutritional tracking, in the knowledge it will provide you when it comes to your additional focus being paid to your diet in terms of food choices and how they contribute towards your macronutrients. You'll know how to effectively track each macronutrient, as laser-focus needs to be on protein, to ensure that you are maintaining lean muscle tissue. For example, during my "on" season, I often choose rice cakes over a tortilla to have with my lean meats. I may also substitute powdered peanut butter for real peanut butter, stick with my low-cal ice cream versus regular ice cream, use artificial sweeteners versus maple syrup or honey, steer clear of unnecessary sauces and/or condiments, and avoid alcohol as much as possible in order to achieve both my TDEE and macronutrient goals.

Although it may be tempting at times during "on" season, especially when you start seeing aesthetic results, to want to be more aggressive with your calorie deficit, you'll understand how this will ultimately contribute to metabolic adaptations. Also, you'll know that you won't want to compromise a higher TDEE that you may have spent time building up over your "off" season, driving your calories down aggressively. You'll know how important it is to remember that the goal during "on" season is to successfully avoid as much metabolic adaptation as possible, keeping your calories as high as possible while still losing body fat. You'll be reminded of how these calories continue to support your effort and goals. Through nutritional tracking, you'll understand how lower levels of TDEEs are very hard to sustain, and they compromise muscle tissue growth and support.

"Maintenance" Season and Intuitive Eating

Through nutritional tracking, you'll understand how "maintenance" season is great in that you can remain at status quo with no intended changes unless you choose, not including the potential stress and efforts of having to gain muscle tissue or lose body fat. You'll be reminded of how it's a good season for the body to just "be" in status quo. . . a mother's long-term goal. Through nutritional tracking, you'll understand how to maintain your TDEE in "maintenance" season by way of your diet and possibly greater movement levels (especially your NEAT levels), while still maintaining your planned resistance training and cardio. This season could last weeks, months, or even years.

With time spent nutritional tracking, a mother will know that after accomplishing successful "on" and "off" seasons, a "maintenance" season is usually entered with a certain kind of mindfulness and a willingness to maintain this status quo. However, she will understand that life still happens and her balance can always be challenged. Muscle tissue may be lost and fat gained over time, which may result in body composition changes. Because it's possible to gain muscle in "maintenance" season as she prioritizes resistance training and practices progressive overload (discussed in a later chapter), she will know how to evaluate weight increases through a body composition test, knowing whether or not she's actually gained weight due to muscle or that she's truly put on body fat. Any calorie surplus or deficit over time, could offset the balance in the maintenance season. A mother's fitness experience will dictate if after a period of time, she will need to enter either an "on" or "off" season again after spending time in their "maintenance" season. Regardless of whether she chooses to or not, she won't fear this transition, as she will enter this new season with confidence in her knowledge of how to track her nutrition with the ReShapeHER program.

Through nutritional tracking, a mother will know how the ebbs and flows of her fitness activity impacts her TDEE and how this may need to be adjusted over time. She may choose to use her techniques of "Intuitive" eating (trusting her body to make food choices for her), to make more of a contribution to her food choices. *In my opinion, Intuitive eating (even for experienced trackers) can be difficult, because this type of eating is hard to sustain in the long run and reach our fitness goals. It can often result in us not obtaining our TDEE and macronutrient requirements, leading us back to nutritional tracking if we want to see consistency in our fitness journey. However, even though Intuitive eating may be difficult to maintain for some, it can serve as a great short-term practice for a mother who needs a break from tracking or long-term for a mother that is an experienced tracker and feels confident in her intuitive choices.*

"Weekly Spread" Approach

Tracking in general and regardless of season, is best done when you can think of it in terms of a "weekly spread." What I mean by this is that you will take your TDEE and multiply it by seven (the number of days in a week) to give you a weekly, calorie number. After doing this, you can spread this number out throughout the week, depending on how you'd like in order to account for lower and higher calorie days or possibly allow for more calories over the weekends (which tend to be days that can derail many people's fitness and nutritional goals). This can be especially helpful for mothers, as it can often be easier to achieve fitness goals while their children are in school or daycare and harder to accomplish on the weekends when they have less time and are consumed with being moms!

An example of a sample week for a typical person that has a daily TDEE of, let's say, 2,000 calories (a weekly average of 14,000), and would like to conserve some calories for their weekends, would look something like the following chart:

TOTAL WEEKLY CALORIES:

Monday	1800 calories
Tuesday	1800 calories
Wednesday	1800 calories
Thursday	1800 calories
Friday	2000 calories
Saturday	2400 calories
Sunday	2400 calories
WEEK TOTAL	14,000 calories

So, you can see that the weekly average will still be 14,000 calories but they are distributed unevenly and in a way that makes sense in order to conserve more calories on the weekend. Personally, this is one of the greatest ways I've been able to achieve my fitness goals and still maintain a social life on the weekends! After all, your social life shouldn't have to suffer because of your fitness goals. This is one of the areas in which the ReShapeHER program understands this and gives you insight as to how you can have the best of both worlds—a great fitness plan in addition to a healthy social life as a mom!

Planning your macronutrients in terms of a weekly spread also steers you away from thinking about incorporating "cheat meals" into your program. I don't believe in cheat meals and here's why: "Cheat" insinuates just that... "cheating." Why would you want to "cheat" yourself from getting results with the nutritional part of your fitness plan? Because here's the thing: If you eat in a surplus, you'll gain weight; if you eat in a deficit, you'll lose weight. Remember, calories are KING (or in our case, QUEEN) when it comes to fat loss, and eating more than you need to consume will derail you from having fat loss success.

However, I understand the need to have a meal that is perhaps untracked or heavier in calorie content to break the monotony. This untracked meal is better accomplished in a "maintenance" or "off" season, as you wouldn't be so concerned with having fat loss results. However, if your goal is fat loss, you should pay more attention to your weekly spread of calories and try to save more for the time of the week that you plan to eat in calorie excess. That way, you can still achieve success even when accounting for a day or so of higher-calorie meals. What tracking allows you to do is to plan for the higher-calorie meals versus "cheating." It puts YOU in the control seat of your choices, and this is a healthy place to be! Also, nutritional tracking helps to not lend to the idea that certain foods should be demonized and may be considered "cheat" foods. It allows you to include everything in your diet as long as it fits within your nutritional goals.

Intermittent fasting (the practice of setting an eating window for a specified period of time each day), is also a technique mother may choose to practice in order to assist her in controlling her daily caloric intake. *(There are other possible benefits to this practice that I won't discuss in this book when it comes to intermittent fasting, as it is mentioned for the sake of discussing a daily caloric spread).* Many like to think of this practice like it's a special diet, but really what it boils down to, is a practice that takes advantage of a non-consumption of calories over a given period of time in the day. When a mother gets used to consuming calories only during a certain eating window it may allow her the ability to consume less calories overall, on any given day. However, intermittent fasting is very individualized and may not provide these results, as the calories consumed during this period of time may end up being higher, considering the body's response to fasting.

There are many other types of techniques that mothers may choose when it comes to controlling her daily caloric consumption. She may choose to skip a meal entirely, choose to make a specific meal a lower-calorie one, avoid calorie intake prior to bedtime or after waking, etc. Regardless of the technique, the outcomes are very individualized and comes down to the fact that calories reign supreme when it comes to a mother's fitness outcomes. An overconsumption of calories over time will lead to weight gain and an underconsumption of calories over time will lead to weight loss.

When it comes to a successful nutritional plan like the one in the ReShapeHER program, it is critical to remember that it needs to incorporate all of the things that support your nutritional requirements as well as provide you the energy to practice your fitness plan. Understanding the quality of what you eat, and how much, is key when reaching your fitness goals and avoiding the yo-yo dieting pitfalls. Nutritional tracking gives you the ability to not only control your fitness seasons you are in with confidence, but also your overall fitness outcomes as they relate to your diet. Remember, you can't outsmart a bad diet! Your nutrition could be the one thing holding you back from reaching your goals in a short period of time. This is why the ReShapeHER program includes nutritional guidelines that you can have confidence in, as you continue in your fitness journey.

CHAPTER 8 CLIFF NOTES

- Macronutrient trackers are great tools in that they allow for you to input the foods that you are consuming on a daily basis in order to understand how they are contributing towards your TDEE and macronutrient goals.
- Once you begin tracking your macronutrients, you'll start to understand how much of each macronutrient you'll need to achieve your goal from not only a plating perspective but also that of a volume one.
- Tracking is best accomplished when it is thought of in terms of a "weekly spread" (amount of calories that can be divided up over the week versus over just a day). This allows mothers more freedom to be more strict on weekdays and possibly save their calories for days (like weekends) in which they may consume more.
- How a mother controls her caloric intake is very individualized.
- Nutritional tracking can put a mother in the control seat of her choices. It doesn't lend to the demonetization of certain foods that may be considered "cheat" foods, but rather allows mothers to include everything in her diet as long as it fits within her nutritional goals.
- Your total macronutrient percentages for the day may fall outside of your ideal percentages and this is fine! Through nutritional tracking, you can learn how to drive these percentages closer to where they need to be over time.

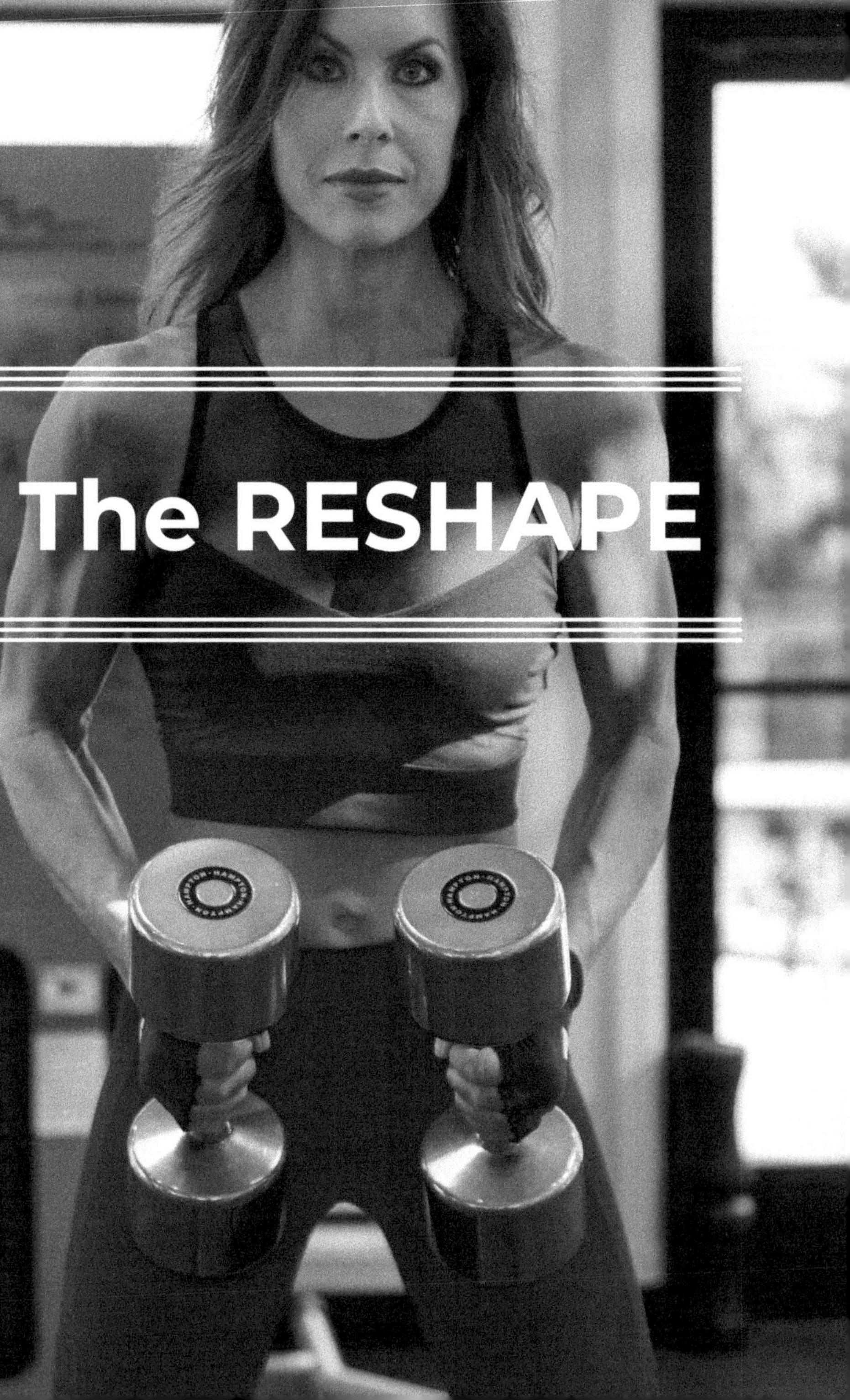

The RESHAPE

9

Combating Pitfall #3

–Muscle Loss

RESISTANCE TRAINING IS ONE OF the most critical components of a fitness plan, in that it is essential to maintaining and developing lean muscle tissue, which along with body fat loss, will be the two biggest contributors to a better body composition and great tone. This is why the ReShapeHER program places a large emphasis on resistance training as part of the overall fitness portion of the plan, making it the priority of any planned workout. As with any new fitness plan, it is critical for all mothers to always consult with their healthcare provider before starting.

Resistance training can improve our movement control, our balance, functional independence, cognitive abilities and self esteem, all of which are of critical importance for a mother. It is an activity that greatly contributes to our overall wellness.

When it comes to resistance training programs, protocols are usually set based on training goals. In the ReShapeHER program, the training protocols that this program includes, will support mothers who desire to achieve a healthy body composition and maintenance and/or grow their lean muscle tissue. This program can be tailored to mothers who want to use it for general health purposes, to mothers who would like to adjust the program variables to support more challenging and specific fitness goals.

Muscle Loss

Resistance training is often avoided by many mothers, resulting in failed fitness attempts because of their lack of contribution to their lean muscle tissue. This avoidance of resistance training results in an overall lack of tone and worsens a mother's overall body composition over time. As a mother ages, this lack of muscle tone is easily blamed on hormones or the aging process, when in fact, it is a direct result of little attention being placed on a mother's muscle tissue. The ReShapeHER program places resistance training as a top priority, helping a mother avoid the fitness detriments of muscle loss. Along with a great nutritional component, this program helps a mother achieve her fitness goals in a short period of time.

The "Bulky" Misconception

Many women tend to avoid resistance training because of the many misconceptions that exist about it, specifically the fear that many women have about getting too "bulky." They tend to prioritize scale weight over understanding their body composition, which takes into account the contributions they are making towards their lean muscle tissue and body fat. They also lack the understanding of how to achieve muscle growth through a successful "off" season, followed by achieving body fat loss through a successful "on" season with nutritional and fitness practices like the ones incorporated in the ReShapeHER program. Because of this, women tend to revert to doing mostly cardiovascular activities to try and achieve their body composition goals. What they find is they can't seem to achieve the lean muscle tone that they'd like with their bodies. With unsuccessful practices, their bodies don't become stronger over time, but rather fatigued and weak from contributing to movements that improve their cardiovascular health but aren't good contributors to their lean muscle tissue.

Should mothers prioritize strength training over just weight loss (which is often depicted by a uni-dimensional measurement such as a house scale), this would lend to them having a bigger difference in how they look and feel in the long run. Five pounds of muscle gain can look vastly different (and often much better) than five pounds of fat loss on a woman's body. Ultimately, continued education is needed when it comes to resistance training and the many benefits it can provide women and mothers. It is critical for women to adopt a plan that incorporates resistance training movements such as the ones suggested in the ReShapeHER program, to ensure that she's making the most out of her strength training efforts and achieving her fitness goals.

Many women fall victim to not understanding how to change their body's composition, especially mothers, after experiencing a life-changing event such as having a baby. They have a hard time knowing what to do with their postpartum bodies, as they often have to face problem areas that are new or magnified as a result of the changes their bodies have endured. More often than not, they have more body fat than they did prior to pregnancy and fear adding any weight to their bodies, even if this means lean muscle tissue. They fail to realize that in the long run, this lean muscle tissue will contribute to a much better body composition once they lose this body fat over time, allowing them to regain or even surpass their previous strength and overall tone.

For many mothers, without a solid fitness plan like the ReShapeHER plan that gives a mother an outline to achieve her best body composition, the thought of trying to regain the body she once had seems overwhelming. Accomplishing these efforts may seem even more overwhelming, knowing they will now have to be accomplished while taking care of a newborn. Because of these things in combination with an overall lack of fitness education, a mother may succumb to the idea that she will always be stuck with a particular problem area or body after pregnancy forever. Or even worse, she may resort to taking a risky approach in combating it through a medical procedure such as a tummy tuck or liposuction. These procedures may make a marked difference on a problem area, yet they still don't address how she can achieve a healthy overall body composition over her lifetime. Without a solid fitness education, a mother can regain body fat, losing the results of what was once achieved through these types of surgeries. She may have been able to avoid these types of surgeries altogether by practicing a solid fitness plan like ReShapeHER that helped her combat these problem areas and reach her fitness goals.

After pregnancy, in order to achieve an ideal body composition, it is critical that a woman understands that this process boils down to her efforts in achieving a healthy balance of muscle tissue and body fat. This balance is what will yield the tone and aesthetic results she desires. Since the body endures many changes during pregnancy, body composition therefore changes, requiring a mother to make an effort to regain a healthy balance of muscle and body fat once again. A mother's efforts to achieve this healthy ratio must be supported with not only a great fitness plan but also a great nutritional plan (both of which are included in the ReShapeHER program).

As I mentioned in a previous chapter, when it comes to trying to achieve fat loss, if every fitness plan was just focused on doing movements that only focused on calorie output in order to achieve an ideal body composition, muscle development wouldn't be made but rather lost over time. This type of plan results in an overall loss of tone. This type of plan also works against us as we grow older, because we lose muscle tone as we age, and this is compounded by focusing primarily on fat loss versus a combination of this and muscle maintenance or growth.

Why Mothers Need to Resistance Train

Without the support of our lean muscle tissue, especially as women and mothers, we subject our bodies to being weaker over time and less able to support the weight of our bodies, resulting in bone loss and injuries. Mothers are especially at risk for not having enough lean muscle tissue, as during pregnancy and after having children, they need additional support to endure not only their own body weight but also that of their offspring. This makes it even more critical for mothers to recognize the importance of supporting their muscle through resistance training with a solid plan incorporated in the ReShapeHER program.

Developing one's body composition takes patience and time. It not only involves fat loss efforts but also that of muscle maintenance and/or growth. As mothers, we need to respect this process and the time it takes, just as we would carrying a baby to full term. Muscle development (otherwise known as hypertrophy) is a complex set of events that allows the muscle to meet the demands we place on it in terms of exercise or function-induced stress.

According to Lyle McDonald (in an article written by M. Matthews at Legion), a health and fitness researcher and writer who has had one-on-one experience helping thousands of people build muscle and lose fat, Lyle found through his research that muscle gain can be categorized by years of proper training. He estimates that women who have properly trained for one year can gain around one pound of muscle per month. Two years of training would result in 0.5 pounds per month, and at three years and beyond, muscle gain can be quite negligible in that there is a rate of diminishing returns. These are the women who have been lifting for many years and have to work harder at making a marked difference in their muscle growth. However, when it comes to this growth, it is important to note that without proper training, these gains can be lost if resistance training efforts aren't continued.[24]

Women in general, also have shorter muscle fibers as well as significantly less muscle tissue, which account for strength differences when compared to men. However, research has shown that neither age nor gender can affect muscle volume response to whole-body strength training. According to the National Institute of Health in their article that evaluated muscle size responses to strength training with a small participant group (eight young men ages 20-30, six young women ages

20-30, and nine older men ages 65-75 as well as a similar group of 10 older women), muscle response and growth as compared to all groups was minimal over a six-month period of time.[25] Nevertheless, even when this response and growth are considered, it is critical to understand that as a woman, a good fitness plan that allows for consistent resistance training is necessary for this muscle response and growth.

Compound Lifts Are Priority

The ReShapeHER program gives a mother an outline for many of the Compound lifts she can do to strengthen the muscle in her common problem areas. These lifts will strengthen a woman's body by using more than one muscle group at a time. This will allow her to train multiple muscle groups at a time, be more efficient in her efforts in building her muscle strength as they require more muscle recruitment to accomplish, and possibly burn more energy in doing so. The ReShapeHER program also includes suggested Isolation lifts that will assist her in zoning in on specific muscle groups and assist her in sculpting her body, along with a nutritious diet. Both of these types of lifts can be done at home or in the gym.

It is critical that the Compound exercises are prioritized first, as they engage more muscle groups and require more energy to accomplish. Accomplishing these lifts first allows a mother to use her energy towards lifts that engage more of her muscle fibers and do them with proper form. Isolation exercises target the specific muscle group you are trying to grow or maintain. One of the keys to remember in preventing injury, is to always ensure that lifts are done with good form. Doing Compound exercises first, will help a mother maintain good form with the energy she puts forth when doing these lifts that involve multiple muscle groups.

Progress with Resistance Training

As a woman continues her resistance training over time, she can choose to use different variations of the lifts that are suggested in this program. She can change the frequency, intensity, rest between sets, etc. of the lifts in the ReShapeHER program as she continues with her fitness journey. It will be important to challenge her body with her routine as she progresses, in order to avoid metabolic adaptation (see Chapter 11 on "Progressive Overload"). This process is very personalized to every individual. Just like nutrition, it is critical for a mother to take notes on her fitness progress to ensure that she knows when adjustments should be made.

There are many other types of other effective, resistance training lifts that are not mentioned in the ReShapeHER program. However, the lifts suggested in this program were chosen because of their effectiveness in targeting the specific muscle groups mentioned in this program and have served instrumental in helping me quickly achieve my ultimate body composition after pregnancy in little time. Should a mother choose to incorporate a lift not mentioned in this program, she can do so, following the protocols included in this program, (such as the times she'll practice the lift every week, the frequency and also following the principles of Progressive Overload, etc).

WORKOUT TIPS FOR SAFETY AND INJURY PREVENTION:

The ReShapeHER program suggests some workout tips below, that will support a mother having a safe workout and hopefully help her prevent injuries along her journey:

1. It is important for mothers to begin every resistance training workout with a warm-up. Warm-ups are suggested to be at least a few minutes or so, including something a mother enjoys doing (like a stationary bike or treadmill walk) to get the blood flowing.

2. It is always important for mothers to do exercises in which they feel stable or familiar versus ones that they feel unstable and unfamiliar, until they advance in their fitness ability. Second, it is critical to start with lighter weights before progressing to heavier ones (see chapter on "Progressive Overload"). Third, it is import-

ant to make sure a lift is accomplished in a slower fashion before doing it too quickly and risking injury. Lastly, I'll mention that this is an area that a mother may want to consider hiring a certified personal trainer in the beginning, to help them understand how to execute resistance training lifts effectively to prevent a future injury. Oftentimes we may think we are executing lifts with good form, when in actuality, we may not be.

3. After a resistance training workout, a mother should take a few minutes to cool-down and do a few static stretches. This should include stretches in which she is standing, sitting or lying still and challenging the muscle groups she focused on in her workout. For example, for a leg day, she could do a simple quad stretch against a wall or a lunge stretch.

4. It is important for a mother to stay well fed and hydrated to support her resistance training efforts. This is not only critical before a workout, but also after a workout, when her body is in need of calorie and hydration replenishment.

5. Lastly, for preventing injury, to improve our range of motion with resistance training and for overall health, it is critical that as mothers, we continue to incorporate flexibility practices into our fitness routines. The ReShapeHER program suggests a mother incorporates some flexibility exercises into her training routine at least two times per week. This can include activities such as basic stretching, yoga, etc.

TRUSTING THE PROCESS

Too often, we give up our resistance training too quickly when we don't see instantaneous results. We need to appreciate that we aren't just making a uni-dimensional contribution toward body fat loss, but rather a multi-dimensional one consisting of muscle maintenance and/or growth in addition to it. Every day that we successfully dedicate ourselves to this process, we make another step toward having the body composition we desire. These steps will collectively add up to future aesthetic results. We need to have patience and a respect for the process, understanding that we can't judge these steps individually but rather as a whole when it comes to accessing our resistance training progress.

With that said, it's critical to remember the "Principle of Variation" when it comes to any workout program. People respond differently to the same program, just as they can respond differently to the same nutritional plan. It is important to remember that like nutrition, we can't compare our progress and outcomes to others as we are all different. The key with any desired outcome, is ensuring that we are being consistent in our practices. Whether it takes us a slower or faster period of time to make the same progress as someone else, doesn't matter. What matters is that we are headed in the direction of our goal, and through our dedication to consistency, we know we'll eventually achieve it.

All of the suggested resistance training lifts in the ReShapeHER program for each problem area are listed below each section and can all be found in the QR-coded video at the end of this chapter!

LIFTS FOR PROBLEM AREA #1

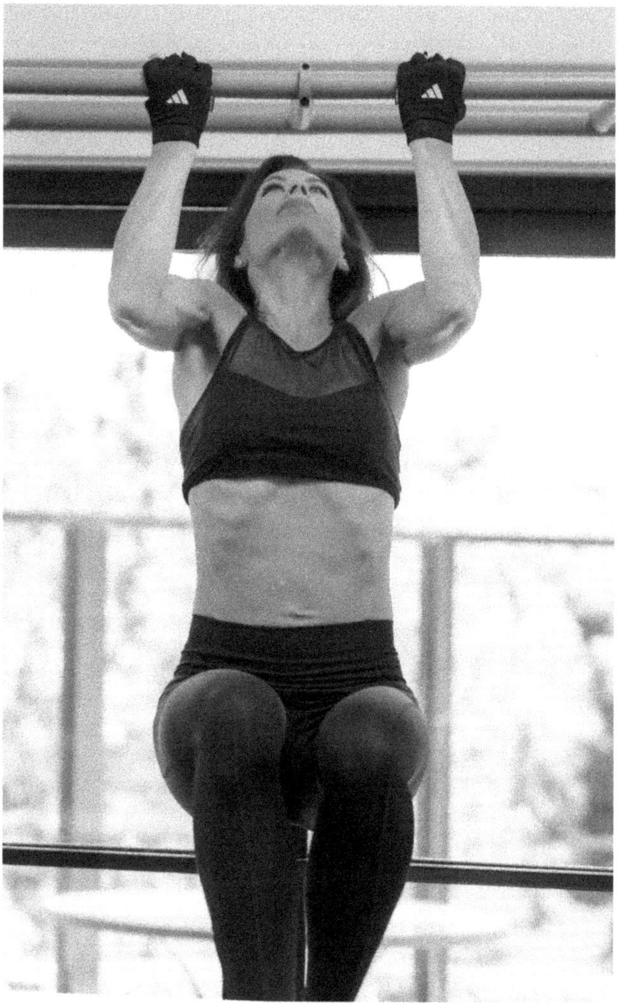

– THE ABDOMINALS

When it comes to a woman engaging the abdominal muscles, unlike other muscle groups, Compound exercises are the best movements to do this. I know from personal experience that I built abs of steel from Compound movements, not from those that strictly isolated my core. Matter of fact, I rarely do isolation exercises to build my abdominal region. Compound lifts work great for the abdominal muscles as they allow them to be natural stabilizers. Isolation movements do not reflect these natural movements. This isn't to say that they can't be done, but it depends on how much growth/hypertrophy you want or need to make in your abdominal area, which is why these lifts are also included in the ReShapeHER program. However, if you want to attack the abs in a time-efficient manner and burn more calories, Compound lifts are the way to go!

The Reason Behind the "Muffin Top"

One area that is a common concern for many mothers is the abdominal region, as it is an area that transforms the most during pregnancy. As the growing uterus stretches the muscles in the mother's abdominal wall, they become susceptible to being weak, torn, split, and damaged. During pregnancy, a mother may have modified everyday core movements that further weakened her core. If this area isn't strengthened prior to pregnancy, it will certainly be much weaker after, further lending to a less-than-optimal tone and body composition in this area. This may result in a woman having the notorious "muffin top" or looking pregnant even after she's had the baby, as a result of her weakened abdominal region.

When it comes to abdominals, it is important to note that every mother's muscles are built differently. Visibly abdominals require a low body fat percentage and can be difficult to achieve for those who may not be genetically blessed to have visible abdominals at these percentages. For many, walking around with a visible six-pack isn't a healthy or sustainable body composition. Regardless of your genetics, achieving toned abdominals can ONLY be accomplished with a solid diet and exercise plan like the ones incorporated in the ReShapeHER program, that allow a mother to achieve a healthy and toned body composition.

The ReShapeHER program incorporates the following Compound and Isolation lifts for the ABDOMINALS:

Compound	Isolation
Suitcase Deadlift	Abdominal Crunches
Medicine Ball Slams (Home Version - can use backpack)	Hanging Knee Raise/Twist (Home Version - can use playground equipment or bar)
Bear Crawl ("moving plank")	Seated Russian Twist
Single-Leg Deadlift	Cable Ab Pulldown (Home Version - "Dumbbell Crunch")

LIFTS FOR PROBLEM AREA #2

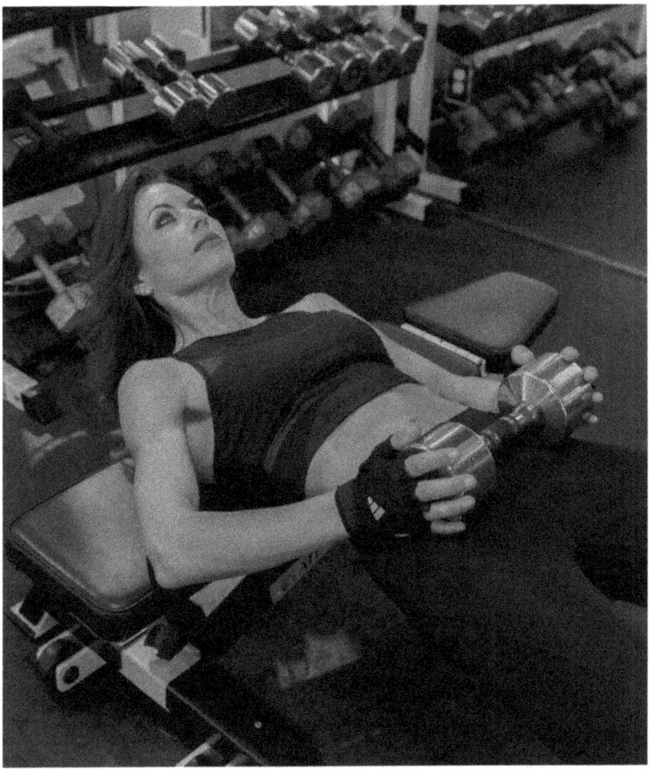

– THE GLUTES

Another problem area for mothers after pregnancy is the glutes region. This is an area that can be affected by hormones, overall body fat gain (as women tend to store fat in this area), and being less active during pregnancy. This is a very frustrating area for many women, postpartum or not. It is often the area that hangs onto body fat the longest and the last to tone up. Matter of fact, it's such a problem area that millennials have even coined the fat that hangs under the buttocks crease, the "banana roll"! Society is always reminding women of the regarded toned and bodacious derriere, especially during summertime bathing suit season. (Maybe we might feel differently if our attire was sought-after swim trunks versus bikinis!)

Nevertheless, the glute region is one that can either be a help or a hindrance for a Mom. The ReShapeHER program addresses this area specifically, giving moms a guide for successful lifts that can target this area and grow or maintain the glutes, in addition to a nutrition guide that allows for body fat reduction. With these two areas being a focus of the ReShapeHER program, body composition can take place and result in toned glutes!

Engaging the Glutes are Key

The beauty about the glutes, in my personal experience, is that you can make drastic changes to them in a short period of time with a good fitness and nutritional plan. The reason for this is they are a larger muscle group that is oftentimes just not being engaged. There's actually some truth to the slang term "lazy butt!" Dormant butt syndrome can happen when glute muscles have forgotten what to do since they haven't been activated properly. This happens when moms haven't incorporated glute exercises into their fitness plans or haven't activated them by sitting for prolonged periods of time, causing the hip flexors to tighten and weaken the glutes.

Oftentimes during pregnancy, it becomes difficult to do many activities that would have otherwise activated the glutes. Combined with a lack of energy during pregnancy, this often results in moms sitting for these prolonged periods of time during pregnancy and thereafter, as they care for their children and go back to work. All of this can be negated by activating the glutes and being consistent with a solid fitness plan like ReShapeHER. This program is designed to combat this problem area as well as provide a nutritional outline to support a mom's effort in doing this.

The ReShapeHER program incorporates both Compound and Isolation lifts that target all three of the muscles that make up the glutes: the gluteus maximus, gluteus medius, and gluteus minimus. Unlike the abdominal muscles, the glutes respond very well to both Compound and Isolation movements, which is why they are included in this successful fitness plan.

By targeting these three muscles with Compound and Isolation exercises, the entire gluteal region can be activated and allow for a toned tush that even combats the all-too-familiar "banana roll." So moms, you can say goodbye to a saggy, untoned, or ill-defined butt and hello to buns of steel with ReShapeHER!

The ReShapeHER program incorporates the following Compound and Isolation lifts for the GLUTES:

Compound	Isolation
Back Squats (Home Version - "Dumbbell Squat")	Hip Thrust (Home Version - "Dumbbell Hip Thrust")
Sumo Deadlifts (Home Version - "Dumbbell Sumo Deadlift")	Cable Kick-backs (Home Version - use Resistance Band)
Bulgarian Split Squats	Hip Abduction/Adduction (Home Version - use Resistance Band
Weighted Step-ups	Reverse Glute Hyper Machine (Home Version - floor)

LIFTS FOR PROBLEM AREA #3

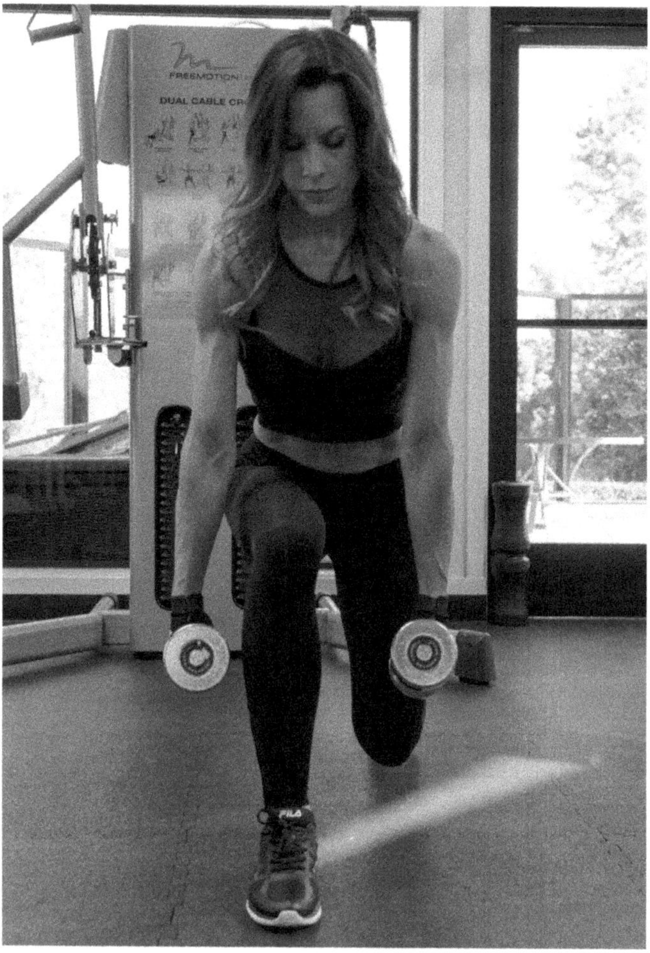

– THIGHS/HAMSTRINGS

In addition to the glutes and abdominal muscles, another problem area for mothers is also the thighs and hamstring region. This area, in addition to the glutes, can tend to carry a lot of cellulite as women tend to store fat in this area. It can oftentimes, along with the glutes, be one of the areas that is the last to tone up, especially if you're a female who tends to carry your weight in your lower body, which is why the nutritional part of the ReShapeHER program will also be key with this area, in addition to resistance training.

Managing Cellulite and "Saddlebags"

One of the biggest annoyances for any mother is the dimpled and lumpy skin many of us have to deal with. It can often become our biggest enemy, especially around bathing suit season and can be the reason why we tend to favor dark colored lycra during other times of the year. There are many factors that cause it that we can't control, like our skin structure, genetics, age and hormones. This can be really frustrating, as some women can suffer from it when others do not. Also, some women can be really thin and actually have more than women that are heavier. The thighs and hamstrings are notorious for carrying these dimples and making it difficult for moms to feel confident in toning these areas.

With all that said, there are ways that mothers can improve, or even control, their cellulite with the ReShapeHER program. Eating a balanced diet, exercising and maintaining a healthy weight are some of the most effective ways it can be managed, and are all supported with this program. When a mother understands what she should be eating, and how much, she can follow a balanced diet. She can put her best efforts towards her exercise, when she understands which movements will contribute to her best body composition, And, she can also maintain a healthy weight by doing all both of these things. The ReShapeHER program gives her the ability to effectively tone her thighs and hamstrings, as well as work towards warding off the cellulite!

The ReShapeHER program incorporates the following Compound and Isolation lifts for the THIGHS AND HAMSTRINGS:

Compound	Isolation
Romanian Deadlift	Seated/Lying Leg Curls (Home Version - use Resistance Band)
Alternating Weighted Step-Ups	Cable Side Leg Raises (Home Version - use Resistance Band)
Walking Lunges	Cable Pull-throughs (Home Version - use Resistance Band)
Leg Press (Home Version - use Resistance Band)	Monster Band Walk

LIFTS FOR PROBLEM AREA #4

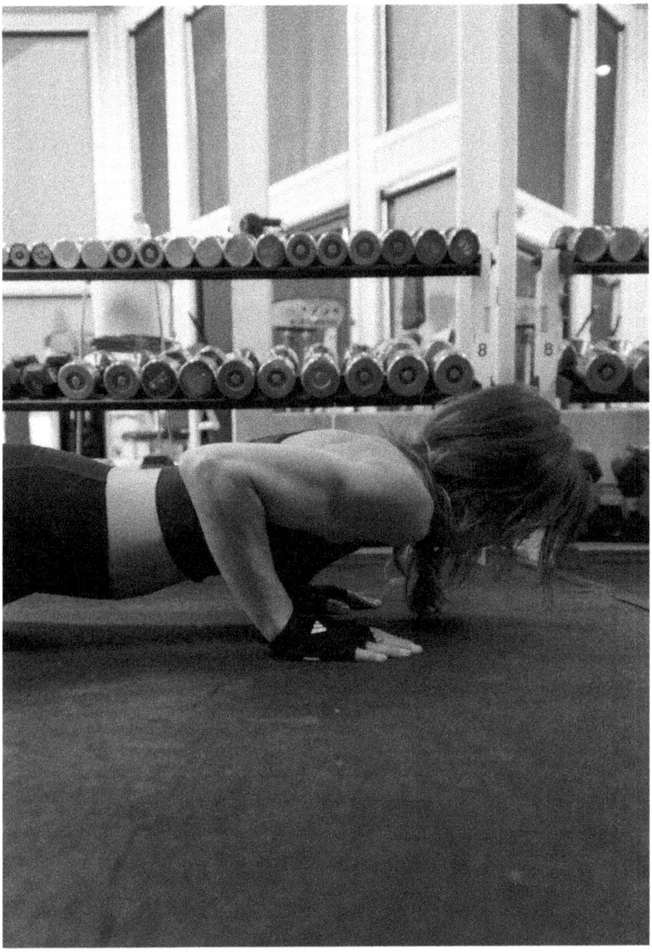

– THE UPPER BODY (ARMS/SHOULDERS/BACK)

The ReShapeHER program addresses a final problem area for mothers - the upper body. This upper body section is divided into three primary areas: shoulders, arms, and back. These areas bring a lot of frustration for women in that they tend to lose tone during pregnancy. Without a successful fitness plan and nutritious diet, they can often end up looking flabby. This can be especially frustrating for moms as these areas typically can't be covered and are especially exposed during warmer months of the year with form-fitting tops, tanks, and bathing suits.

Many mothers, due to hormonal fluctuations, can tend to have a warmer body temp and may want to sport these types of summer clothes throughout the year, which makes the situation even worse if they feel like their body tone in these areas doesn't support their comfort in doing so. They start to notice the bulges in areas they didn't before: the fat rolls near their bra straps, back fat, and the coined "bat wings" that seem to flap every time they might wave goodbye to a friend. The good news is that these are all areas the ReShapeHER program allows a mom to attack head-on, with a solid fitness plan that incorporates resistance training.

Many of the Compound exercises mentioned above that you will be executing for the other muscle groups, will also be strengthening the shoulders, arms, and back. For example, the deadlift, which is an amazing exercise for the glutes and legs, will also require muscle recruitment from the arms, which in turn will also help strengthen this area. Therefore, when this program is fully completed each week, no muscle group will be left out. All of the lifts will work in harmony to create a tight and toned body for any mother who consistently completes it!

The "X-Factor"

The ReShapeHER program is designed to sculpt the female body. This plan understands and supports the uniqueness of the hourglass shape or "X factor." This hourglass or X shape is achieved by having nicely defined shoulders and arms (top of the X shape), a tight back and small waist (the middle of the X), and strong glutes (the bottom of the X). All of these things combined creates this coveted hourglass shape that is aesthetically appealing.

The ReShapeHER program takes this into consideration, in that it includes lifts to tighten and grow the shoulders in this section, which many women neglect, as they don't understand that this creates the very strong top of the "X." By defining the shoulders and arms, it also gives the illusion of a smaller waist. Additionally, tight and defined shoulders and arms can also give the illusion of a smaller lower body if you happen to be heavier in this area. By growing and defining the shoulders and arms, as well as tightening the abdominal wall and lower body with this program, mothers can successfully achieve this highly revered hourglass shape.

The ReShapeHER Program incorporates the following Compound and Isolation lifts for the SHOULDERS, ARMS and BACK:

	SHOULDERS	ARMS	BACK
Com-pound	Overhead Press	Pull-Up and Chin-Ups (Home Version - use playground equipment or bar)	Bent-Over Barbell Row (Home - "Bent-over Dumbbell Row")
	Push Up	Barbell Curl ("Dumbbell Curl")	V-Grip Lat Pulldown (Home - "Upright Dumbbell Row")
		Cable Press-downs (Home Version- "Tricep Dips")	Inverted Row (Home Ver-sion - use low bar or table)
		Kettlebell Swings (Home Version - "Overhead Dumbbell Swing")	

Isolation	Single-Arm Front Raise	Single-Arm Dumbbell Curls	Single-Arm Seated Cable Row (Home Version - use Resistance Band)
	Single-Arm Lateral Raise	Single-Arm Tricep Pushdowns (Home - "Tricep Kickbacks")	Single-arm Lat Pulldown (Home Version - "Dumbbell Inverted Row")
			Straight-arm Cable Pulldown (Home Version - use Resis-tance Band)

RESISTANCE TRAINING – PUTTING IT ALL TOGETHER

When it comes to incorporating resistance training into a fitness plan, there are critical things that need to be taken into consideration prior to doing so. First, if a mother is planning to do all of her planned exercise (EAT) in one session, resistance training should be considered as the first priority in her session over cardiovascular activities on days when both are planned for any given day. The reason for this is because resistance training is critical to developing and maintaining lean muscle tissue, which will be the biggest contributor to a fit body composition. Most importantly, by doing resistance training first, it allows a mother to reserve her energy to contribute not only to maximizing the amount of energy she can contribute to her lifts but also allows her to have the energy reserve to conduct her lifts with good form, preventing injury as a result.

When doing resistance training, it is important to remember that in order to achieve long-term success, a mother needs to practice a fitness plan that incorporates it not only for muscle maintenance and/

or growth, but also for overall strength and injury prevention. This is one of the reasons why the ReShapeHER program is a solid program for mothers to achieve this!

The Mind-Muscle Connection

A critical area to consider when a mother is trying to achieve optimal body composition through her muscle maintenance and growth, as well as preventing injury, is possibly achieved through her mind-muscle connection. It is necessary for a mother to remember to make a mind-muscle connection when doing lifts for each muscle group. According to Bodybuilding.com, through the synaptic connections that can be made between mind and muscle, a woman is not only able to target specific muscle groups but also make the most out of her workout in terms of her hypertrophy (muscle growth).[26]

What the mind-muscle connection means is that you are going to focus on your body as it moves and make a mental connection to the muscle group you are working. For example, when doing a lift for your abdominals, you are going to think about feeling these muscles. You will ask yourself, "Are they engaged?" "How do I know this?" "Can I feel or see them moving?" "How does this movement feel?"

If you sense that an MMC is not being achieved, you will need to focus more intently on the muscle group being isolated or choose another movement that gives a better engagement. Isolation lifts allow you to focus more specifically on muscle groups as they target them; however, it is also important to focus on the muscle group you'd like to target with compound lifts even though other muscle groups are being engaged. Practicing a good mind-muscle connection with specific muscle groups will allow for better potential growth as the engagement of these groups is more likely if an M-M-C is made.

The Importance of Good Form

In addition to performing resistance training first and keeping a good mind-muscle connection, exercising proper form and technique is critical when a mother wants to have successful results and also prevent injury with her resistance training. It is always important to remember that form should trump any type of weight that you are able to lift. Lifting lighter weights with proper form is always better than lifting heavier weights with poor form. Proper form is also the starting point that is required before initiating any type of Progressive Overload (as I'll discuss in the next chapter).

Although there is always a chance of injury to occur even with our best efforts, as mothers we can put our best foot forward by performing resistance training first, performing it with a great mind-muscle connection and also with great form. Lastly, building one's strength up gradually (the "low and slow" technique) by incorporating the science of Progressive Overload (of which I'll discuss in the next chapter) will also prevent injury and lend to long-term results.

Determining Your Number of Repetitions and Sets

When it comes to how much time will be spent on each resistance training exercise, as well as how many of these can fit into each planned session, this will be dictated by the number of sets and reps you do for each one. Your reps (or "repetitions") is the number of times you complete a full exercise movement, while your sets will be the number of times you complete your total number of repetitions as determined by your fitness goal. For example, an average suggestion for a specific lift would be about 10-12 repetitions for three sets. How you accomplish your sets and reps will be based on your fitness goal. According to the American Council of Exercise, reps and sets are recommended based on training goals. There are four goals: Endurance, Muscle Definition, Maximum Strength, and Power. (It is italicized under their chart that for best results, the last rep should achieve momentary fatigue, 30).

If a mother's goal is endurance, their number of repetitions would be equal to or less than 12. For muscle definition, the rep range is 8-15. For maximum strength, it is no greater than (or equal to) six. For power, it highlights explosive barbell lifts as an example, with a rep range of

1-2, and also jumps/medicine ball throws with a rep range of less than eight. *The ReShapeHER program suggests a rep range for mothers, that focuses on muscle definition in order to achieve her optimal body composition. In this case, the rep range suggested is anywhere from 8-15 according to ACE.*[27] *The ReShapeHER program also recommends a rest period of 1-2 minutes between the lower-intense exercises with light loads and 2-3 minutes for higher-intense exercises that use heavier loads, as suggested by ACE.*

When it comes to sets, according to ACE, "a client new to resistance training should start with one to two sets per exercise using a slow-to-moderate tempo (3:1:2 to 4:2:3) to recruit the motor units to activate their attached muscle fibers."[28] In their article discussing how to set up the right sets for clients, they also discuss DOMS (delayed onset muscle soreness) and how too much muscle damage with resistance training can be dangerous. They explain how sets can be changed once a client has experienced initial strength gains and has adjusted to the physical demands of a resistance training program. The article states that "three to four sets is generally considered effective for younger, healthy adults seeking aesthetic results from strength training, while one to three sets can be considered optimal for older adults seeking health benefits."

The ReShapeHER program takes into consideration the ACE guidelines for sets and reps [29], *suggesting a beginning goal for a woman at a repetition range of 8-15 reps for 1-2 sets for each lift. As she progresses, the suggestion is that a woman performs each lift at a repetition range of 8-15 for a maximum of 3-4 sets.* Additionally, when she practices the method of Progressive Overload, in order to prevent injury, she may choose to lower her set and/or rep range to accommodate for the increase in weight until she reaches her maximum suggested rep range of 8-15 for 3-4 sets. Any time you begin any new fitness plan, the body needs time to adjust. Starting with low weights and progressing with lower weights to higher weights slowly over time, allows a woman's body to adjust as well as avoid injury.

Other Resistance Training Variables to Consider

There are other variables to consider when resistance training, other than knowing your number of sets and repetitions, that should be included in your planned workout session. These other variables include the tempo (the speed in which you perform each lift), the intensity (the measure of how difficult an exercise is, expressed as a percentage of a 1RPM - 1 rep max) and the time you'll rest in between sets of each lift. For many, this may sound complicated, but it doesn't have to be! I will explain how the ReShapeHER program includes these variables to make it easy for a mother to consider all of these variables to meet her goals.

The ReShapeHER follows recommended ACE guidelines for slow-to-moderate tempo (3:1:2 to 4:2:3), 31. What this means is that a mother is going to perform her lift by lengthening her muscle for 3-4 seconds (eccentric phase), followed by holding her lift for 1-2 seconds (isometric phase), and finally contract her muscle for 2-3 seconds (concentric phase). So for example, when a mother is doing a bent-over barbell row, she will spend 3-4 seconds lowering the bar below her, followed by 1-2 seconds of holding the bar below her with her arms fully extended, and then spending 2-3 seconds pulling the bar towards her midline to complete the lift.

When it comes to the intensity of how each lift is performed, *the ReShapeHER program recommends all mothers start out at 70% 1RPM (1 rep maximum) for beginners. What this means is that a mother will be lifting her weights at 70% of her overall maximum ability, (1RPM means that this equates to 70% of her overall ability for one rep maximum).* A mother can determine this percentage by doing one rep of an exercise and then gauging her effort. If it's easier than 70% of her maximum effort, she would know to add weight. If it's higher than this percentage, she would know that lowering the weight is needed. For a mother that's more experienced, the ReShapeHER program encourages her to do 70-100% 1RPM, (as recommended by the ACSM).[30]

Lastly, when it comes to the time allotted for rest between each set, *the ReShapeHER program follows ACE guidelines in suggesting a 1-2 minute rest for beginners or mothers who are performing lower-moderate intensity exercises and 2-3 minutes for higher intensity exercises.*[31] For example, a mother who is beginning the ReShapeHER Fitness program, would perform a bicep curl at 70% 1RPM and would rest 1-2 minutes between sets versus an experienced mother performing a bicep curl at 85% 1RPM, that would probably require a 2-3 minute rest.

The following chart illustrates the ReShapeHER Fitness Program variable outline for a mother who is a beginner to one who is more advanced:

	BEGINNER	ADVANCED
Repetitions	8-15	8-15
Sets	1-2	3-4
Tempo	3:1:2	4:2:3
Rest Time	1-2 min	2-3 min
1RPM	70-85%	70-100%

All of the resistance training movements for the ReShapeHER program, can be found in the QR code at the end of the chapter. They are all explained and demonstrated in this video for a mother to have at her fingertips, whether she be on a laptop or mobile device. These lifts can be accomplished at home, or in a gym. Should these be done at home, a mother will need to have the following equipment:

ReShapeHER Program Home Equipment Needs
Dumbbells
Medicine Ball or Heavy Duffle Bag
Resistance Bands - looped and open
Sturdy Chair/Table
Hanging Bar (or playground equipment)
Floor mat

The ReShapeHER Resistance Training Video:

Summary

It is important to remember that when practicing any fitness plan, it is critical that it does incorporate a resistance training component. A fitness plan like the ReShapeHER program that includes resistance training along with a nutritional plan, is a successful way for a mother to build a strong and optimal body composition. Continual stress placed on her lean muscle tissue, in addition to providing it the key nutrients in order to maintain and/or grow it, is essential if a woman wants to achieve an ideal physique. Practicing this fitness portion of the ReShapeHER program with patience and consistency will be the driving components for a mother to yield herself exponential muscle growth and better overall tone. Through these practices, a mother can also successfully combat muscle loss. When it comes to a mother's overall fitness, by practicing the ReShapeHER program, she will ultimately develop healthy fitness habits that can lend to the betterment of her overall health.

With a simple click, you will have all of the ReShapeHER resistance Training lifts and information about them, at your fingertips on your laptop or mobile device.

CHAPTER 9 CLIFF NOTES:

- It is critical for all mothers to always consult with their healthcare provider before starting any new workout program or modifying an existing one.
- Resistance training is one of the most critical components of a fitness plan, in that it is essential to maintaining and developing lean muscle tissue, which along with body fat loss, will be the two biggest contributors to a better body composition and great tone.
- Many women tend to avoid resistance training because of the many misconceptions that exist about it, resulting in failed fitness attempts.
- Women tend to revert to doing mostly cardiovascular activities to try and achieve their body composition goals, resulting in weakness and fatigue as a result of their efforts not contributing to the maintenance or development of their lean muscle tissue.
- Developing one's body composition takes patience and time. It not only involves fat loss efforts but also that of muscle maintenance and/or growth.
- The ReShapeHER program gives a mother an outline for compound lifts she can do to strengthen her muscle by using one or more muscle group at a time, in addition to isolation lifts that will assist her in zoning in on specific muscle groups, allowing her to further sculpt her body. Compound lifts should be accomplished first, as they require more energy as they involve more muscle groups and muscle fiber recruitment.
- The ReShapeHER program includes both compound and isolation resistance training lifts to target four, potential problematic areas for a mother's body: abdominal region, the glutes, thighs/hamstrings and the upper body (specific to shoulders, arms, and back).

- There are many variations of the lifts mentioned in the ReShapeHER program and these can all be done at home or in the gym. For home workouts, minimal equipment is required to accomplish the lifts in all of the four problem areas addressed in this program:

ReShapeHER Program Home Equipment Needs
Dumbbells
Medicine Ball or Heavy Duffle Bag
Resistance Bands - looped and open
Sturdy Chair/Table
Hanging Bar (or playground equipment)
Floor mat

The following are the Compound and Isolation lifts recommended in the ReShapeHER program for sculpting a mother's ABDOMINALS.

For abdominals to be visible, it requires a solid diet along with a lower body fat percentage.

Compound	Isolation
Suitcase Deadlift	Abdominal Crunches
Medicine Ball Slams (Home Version - can use backpack)	Hanging Knee Raise/Twist (Home Version - can use playground equipment or bar)
Bear Crawl ("moving plank")	Seated Russian Twist
Single-Leg Deadlift	Cable Ab Pulldown (Home Version - "Dumbbell Crunch")

The following are the Compound and Isolation lifts recommended for sculpting a mother's **GLUTES.**

Making drastic changes to the glutes require targeting and activating the three muscle groups that make up the glutes.

Compound	Isolation
Back Squats (Home Version - "Dumbbell Squat")	Hip Thrust (Home Version - "Dumbbell Hip Thrust")
Sumo Deadlifts (Home Version - "Dumbbell Sumo Deadlift")	Cable Kick-backs (Home Version - use Resistance Band)
Bulgarian Split Squats	Hip Abduction/Adduction (Home Version - use Resistance Band
Weighted Step-ups	Reverse Glute Hyper Machine (Home Version - floor)

The following are the Compound and Isolation lifts recommended for sculpting a mother's **THIGHS and HAMSTRINGS.**

The thighs and hamstrings can be activated with many of the same types of Compound exercises used to activate the glutes.

Compound	Isolation
Romanian Deadlift	Seated/Lying Leg Curls (Home Version - use Resistance Band)
Alternating Weighted Step-Ups	Cable Side Leg Raises (Home Version - use Resistance Band)
Walking Lunges	Cable Pull-throughs (Home Version - use Resistance Band)
Leg Press (Home Version - use Resistance Band)	Monster Band Walk

---

The following are the Compound and Isolation lifts recommended for sculpting a mother's upper body SHOULDERS, ARMS and BACK.

***The shoulder region is an area that many mothers tend to neglect in their fitness plans. By defining the shoulders, arms and back, this can create the illusion of an "X" factor - a toned upper body, smaller waist and a better smaller lower body that all help to create the revered hourglass shape*

	Shoulders	Arms	Back
Com-pound	Overhead Press	Pull-Up and Chin-Ups (Home Version - use playground equip-ment or bar)	Bent-Over Barbell Row (Home - "Bent-over Dumbbell Row")
	Push Up	Barbell Curl ("Dumb-bell Curl")	V-Grip Lat Pulldown (Home - "Upright Dumbbell Row")
		Cable Press-downs (Home Version- "Tricep Dips")	Inverted Row (Home Ver-sion - use low bar or table)
		Kettlebell Swings (Home Version - "Overhead Dumb-bell Swing")	
Isola-tion	Single-Arm Front Raise	Single-Arm Dumbbell Curls	Single-Arm Seated Cable Row (Home Version - use Resistance Band)
	Single-Arm Lateral Raise	Single-Arm Tricep Pushdowns (Home - "Tricep Kickbacks")	Single-arm Lat Pulldown (Home Version - "Dumb-bell Inverted Row")
			Straight-arm Cable Pulldown (Home Version - use Resistance Band)

- Resistance training should be first priority in a fitness session (over cardiovascular activities) on days when both are planned.
- A mind-muscle connection can possibly help a woman achieve an optimal body composition through her muscle maintenance and growth, as well as prevent injury.
- Exercising proper form when resistance training is critical when a mother wants to have successful results and also prevent injury.

	BEGINNER	ADVANCED
Repetitions	8-15	8-15
Sets	1-2	3-4
Tempo	3:1:2	4:2:3
Rest Time	1-2 min	2-3 min
1RPM	70-85%	70-100%

- A fitness plan like the ReShapeHER program that includes resistance training along with a nutritional plan, is the only way for a woman to build a strong and optimal body composition.

The ReShapeHER Resistance Training Video:

bitly

NOTES

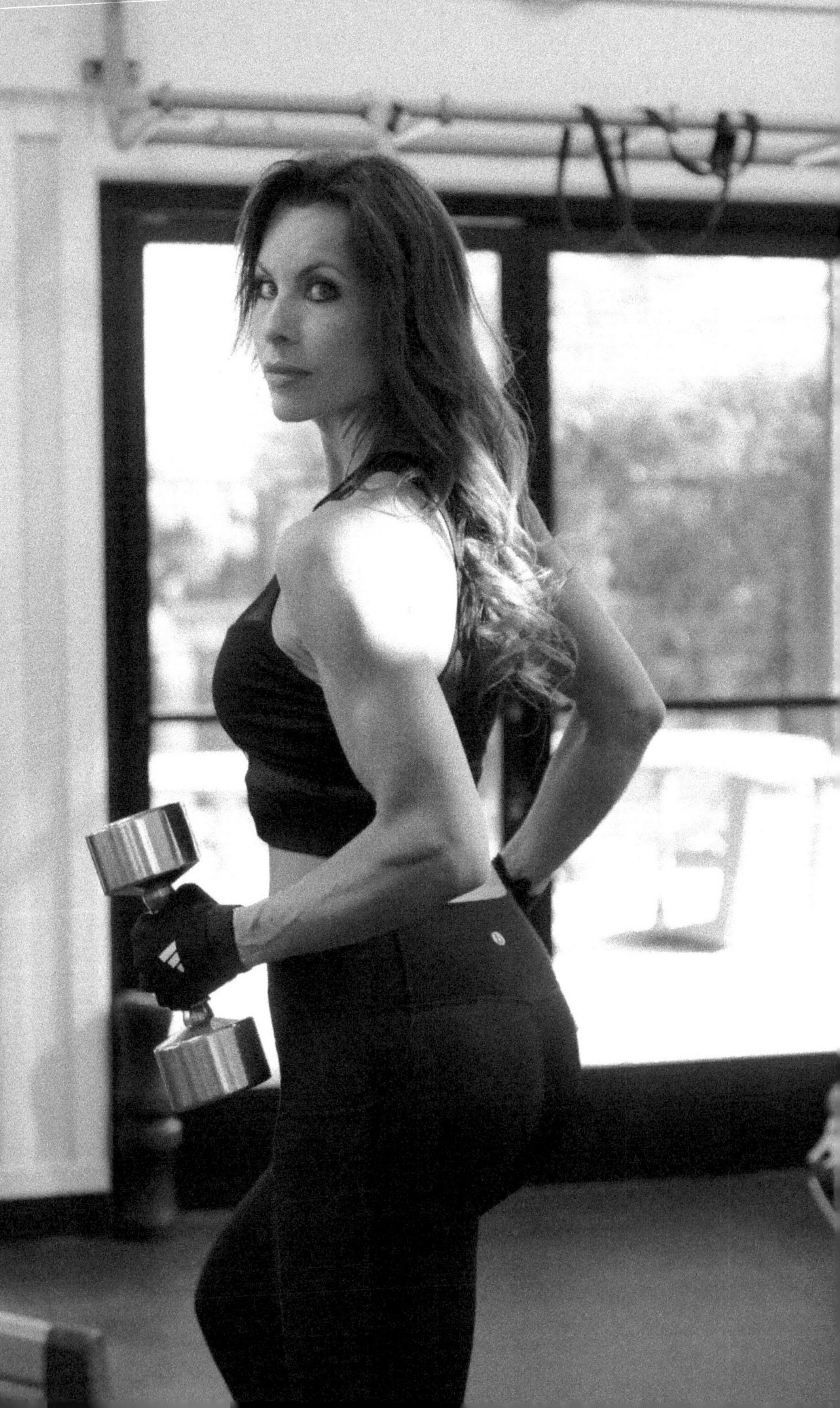

10

Combating Pitfall #4

—Too Much Planned Cardio

MOVEMENT AND EXERCISE ARE INTEGRAL parts of a healthy fitness plan. Physical activity in general, promotes not only strong muscles and bones but also improves respiratory, cardiovascular, and overall health. Staying active and contributing toward your EAT and NEAT helps you possibly maintain a healthy weight, reduce your risk for many diseases and some cancers, and very possibly increase your chances of living longer. When it comes to cardiovascular exercise, it can help improve endurance, oxygen utilization efficiency, and cardiac respiratory function.

Resistance training not only helps muscle growth but also contributes to overall strength, enhances coordination, and helps prevent injury. It is one of the most important pieces of the ReShapeHER Program, as it supports the precious lean muscle tissue that will allow you to have a better body composition over time. As a critical part of our planned exercise (EAT), we cannot overlook the contribution resistance training makes to our overall body composition goals and our overall wellness. I discussed in the previous chapter that without resistance training, a mother will risk losing her lean muscle tissue and therefore suffer when it comes to her body composition.

When utilized appropriately, cardiovascular activities can also make a positive contribution to a fitness plan. These types of movements can also be versatile when it comes to our planned and unplanned exercise and often require little to no equipment. They also help us contribute the most to our calorie output when it comes to reaching our fitness goals as mothers. The ReShapeHER program understands this and incorporates both EAT and NEAT cardio activities successfully to enable a mother to reach her body composition goals.

When it comes to resistance training, however, it can be deceiving when it comes to the amount of calorie output it provides despite the amount of effort it takes to accomplish (although through its ability to develop and support lean muscle tissue, a better metabolism over time may be expected). This is the reason why it's important, not only for cardiovascular health, that cardiovascular exercises are also a part of a successful fitness plan to contribute towards a mother's calorie output. It is important to understand where cardiovascular activities fit into a fitness plan and how to use them to your greatest advantage. Additionally, it is imperative to understand how NEAT (non-exercise activity) plays into this cardiovascular piece of your fitness plan.

Tips for Safety and Injury Prevention

It is important that when performing cardiovascular activities, as with weight training, it is critical that a mother follows the same safety considerations for resistance training, should her cardio be performed alone. She should begin every cardio workout with a quick warm-up. Warm-ups are suggested to be at least around 5 minutes. Additionally, she should do exercises that allow her to feel stable or more familiar at first and then work her way up. For example, a mother beginning a fitness plan shouldn't start out doing high-intensity cardiovascular movements before becoming familiar with lower-intensity ones. A cool-down for about 5 minutes is also suggested with each cardio session. Staying hydrated is also key for both cardiovascular and resistance training, as well as a solid diet that supports her efforts prior to, and after a workout.

Low-intensity, Steady-State Cardiovascular Exercise (LISS)

Low-intensity cardio, otherwise known as LISS, is a type of exercise that allows a mother to keep her heart rate at a comfortable level (typically @50% of its maximum). This type of cardio can be great for mothers after pregnancy, recovering from an injury, etc. It can include things such as walking, light jogging, elliptical machines, going up and down stairs, gardening, shooting baskets, etc. LISS cardio allows a mother to accomplish her movements without the greater amount of effort that she'd have to contribute with higher-intensity exercises, therefore, allowing her to possibly contribute more time to doing them (if she has it). LISS exercises can easily be transitioned to higher intensity ones, by increasing the contribution of effort over 50%. Therefore, these types of exercises can be a great starting point for any mother, or could even be the type of cardio that an advanced mother may choose depending on her time dedication.

High-Intensity, Interval Training (HIIT)

High-intensity cardio, otherwise known as HIIT, can improve cardiovascular health and endurance, as the energy requirement to accomplish these movements are greater than LISS. HIIT can include activities such as jumping jacks, lunges, mountain climbers, push-ups, high knees, rowing, sprints, cycling, etc. The benefit to HIIT cardio, is that the calorie output can be higher in a given amount of time versus LISS cardio. This can be especially beneficial for mothers who want to lose weight and don't have as much time to dedicate to cardio in their schedule. However, it is important to realize that these movements take an incredible amount of energy and will result in more fatigue than LISS. Choosing HIIT over LISS should be made based on a mother's fitness level in order to prevent injury and allow for proper recovery time.

Cardiovascular Activities that Incorporate Resistance Training

There are many types of cardiovascular activities that incorporate both resistance training and cardiovascular movements, that can also be lumped into the HIIT category. One of these types of movements is called "plyometrics". They are technically labeled under cardio because they can raise your heart rate as they are accomplished, however, they are a form of resistance training, in that they boost your muscle power and should follow the same principles of progressive overload (I discuss in the following chapter). Plyometric activities could include such activities as box jumping, split squat jumps, single leg hops, lunge jumps, etc. These types of exercises are great, in that they allow a mother to increase her caloric output in a shorter amount of time, as well as allow for her to develop her muscular performance. These movements can be weaved into an existing resistance-training program and be done in between lifts (with ones requiring more effort done first). These movements should also be chosen based on a mother's fitness level.

When to Practice Cardio with Resistance Training

It is important to note that on days that cardio is to be performed alone and separate from resistance training, cardio should immediately follow resistance training and never be completed prior (unless it is performed another time of the day). This is because a mother will want to dedicate all of her energy in the first part of her workout to her resistance training to ensure that all of her lifts are done safely and with great form. The ReShapeHER program also recommends LISS cardio for its cardio portion for beginners, to ensure that these mothers can allow for enough energy that is required to accomplish their resistance training goals as their bodies adapt to the program. Mothers with more advanced fitness levels can still choose to do HIIT training for their cardio portion of this program.

How to Choose Cardiovascular Activities

The cardiovascular exercise portion of the ReShapeHER program is less important in terms of the type that is done, other than it is done consistently and it is something you enjoy. It is true that if you don't do something you enjoy, you'll cease doing it, which is why it's important to pick 1-2 activities that you will consistently do over time! It is important to understand that with cardio, it may serve as a critical role in terms of your calorie output but isn't as critical as resistance training in terms of how it contributes to the development of lean muscle tissue.

The cardiovascular part of your fitness plan can be enjoyable as a mother, in that you have many different options to choose from. And, choosing different options keeps your fitness environment ever-changing for your body, and helps you avoid metabolic adaptation to any one particular exercise pattern. For example, you could do walking one day and running the next. Maybe one day you do a bike ride and the next day a swim. The great thing is that there are many options when it comes to cardiovascular exercise.

Whether you choose to do HIIT (high-intensity interval training) like running for long distances, sprints or cardio circuits or LIIS (low-intensity steady state) cardio like walks or leisurely bike rides, the same goal can be accomplished in terms of body fat loss. Of course, there are always caveats to this. With lower-intensity cardio, less calorie output is accomplished over a given time period. High-intensity cardio can provide much more in terms of cardiovascular endurance and output, which in turn allows for a greater calorie output and possible contribution to overall body fat loss, which is one of its benefits. However, because HIIT training requires more energy exertion during the same period of time as LIIS, not only can it exhaust the body but it can also contribute to more required recovery time. For this reason, the ReShapeHER program recommends HIIT training for mothers who are more advanced in their fitness levels due to its additional energy requirements. Should a mother choose to practice HIIT for her cardio requirements with the ReShapeHER program, it is best done by allowing her body the time to recover by possibly alternating these sessions with LISS ones throughout the week. However, should a mother decide to do LISS cardio only, she can certainly achieve her fitness and body composition goals. *(I have been able to achieve a successful body composition and compete on stage in Bodybuilding by doing LISS cardio alone!)*

The Phenomenon of "Diminishing Returns"

According to the National Institute of Health, "further exertion of beyond 1 hour of daily cardiovascular exercise produces diminishing returns and may even cause adverse CV effects in some individuals."[32] The phenomenon of diminishing returns is why the ReShapeHER program recommends a minimum of 15 minutes of cardio, in addition to a recommendation of not exceeding 60 minutes of cardio activity, on days where there is a planned cardiovascular exercise component (either proceeding resistance training or done alone). Due to the phenomenon of diminishing returns, the ReShapeHER program includes a time commitment for a mother's cardiovascular exercises (discussed in Chapter 12) to be at a minimum of 15 minutes (with a 60-minute maximum), on days where it is listed alone and also on days listed with resistance training.

The Importance of Rest

Our lifestyles as mothers, our motivation to achieve more with less time, social and emotional pressures, our lack of patience and many other things can often lead us to a place of over-training. Not every mother falls into this category of pushing their bodies with their fitness training beyond their limitations and suffering the consequences, yet a mother that lacks overall rest can often suffer the same consequences. Both can diminish the respect a mother has for her body's boundaries and can lead to many symptoms, such as increased inflammation, a risk for injury or illness, impaired sex hormones, disrupted sleep patterns, appetite and/or mood changes and many other things. This can negate a mother's progress towards her goals, in that these symptoms may derail her energy and efforts, ultimately causing her to fall short of her body composition and health goals.

The importance of rest can often be overlooked and grossly underrated, when it comes to achieving our fitness goals as mothers. Sometimes one of the hardest decisions we can make is listening to our bodies and making a decision to take our feet off the pedal and not accomplish our planned activities for the day. However, sometimes this is necessary in order to recharge and allow our bodies to have the energy to carry out the necessary functions they need to do, in order for us to make fitness progress. Often, with rest comes growth.

If you think about rest in terms of muscle growth, it is imperative in order to build stronger muscles. When you practice resistance training, it creates microscopic tears in your muscle tissue. During rest, your body repairs these tears. Stronger muscles are built through this healing and repair process. Therefore, without rest, this process couldn't take place and we would do the opposite... break muscle down.

Rest is an essential part of any fitness plan. Yet, it doesn't mean you're laying around on the couch all day. Staying active is an essential part of being a fit and healthy mom. Daily movement (or NEAT—non-exercise activity) is still critical, which is why a daily step count of 8,000 steps is included in both the 3-Day and 5-Day ReShapeHER Plans (discussed later in this chapter). However, on rest days, it is important for the body to take breaks from your EAT (planned exercise). This rest allows your body to recover from what you've already accomplished with your routine, prevents muscle fatigue, reduces risk of injury, improves performance and improves sleep.

Metabolic Adaptation

When it comes to cardiovascular activities and their greater contribution to a caloric output versus resistance training, oftentimes mothers tend to put their calorie deficit efforts into overdrive when they want to lose body fat. They often combine this with dieting hard, further contributing to this caloric output. What happens to our bodies when we do this, especially if we do it too frequently without adequate "off" seasons, is that we negatively affect our metabolism. With too many calorie deficits over time, or ones that last too long, our body becomes even better at achieving metabolic adaptation and the ability to survive on these lower numbers of calories. As mothers, not only do we burn ourselves out and end up not being able to keep up with the energy demands with these practices, but we also create a situation that puts our metabolic adaptation into overdrive. This is the reason why many mothers end up in the yo-yo cycle of dieting and perhaps turning into "cardio bunnies" in order to try and achieve their body composition goals. Building a stellar physique takes time. Allowing your body the proper amount of time to build lean muscle tissue, followed by a period of time to effectively lose body fat, is how you reach your body composition goals. This can be successfully accomplished through the ReShapeHER program, by establishing your fitness goals around your fitness "seasons".

Fat Burners

Fat burner supplements are often used by mothers to increase their efforts with calorie expenditure, as they claim to increase fat metabolism, impaired fat absorption, increase weight loss and/or increase fat oxidation during exercise. Unfortunately for some, they work by elevating blood pressure and this can be problematic for those suffering from normal high blood pressure. Most fat burners may also have a high amount of caffeine and other chemicals in them that may be harmful for mothers who aren't privy to reading labels. Manufacturers often promote them as miracle solutions, when in fact, they can often be harmful. When a mother practices the ReShapeHER program consistently, she will not need to take fat burners to achieve results.

NEAT (NON-EXERCISE ACTIVITY THERMOGENESIS)

I discussed in previous chapters the importance of NEAT—your Non-Exercise Activity Thermogenesis and how it makes up 15% of your daily expenditure. Things such as walking, doing household chores, taking stairs versus the elevator, standing versus sitting, and just being "active" all count toward your NEAT expenditure. Your NEAT expenditure is accomplished through your daily movements and is categorized as unplanned exercise, yet contributes a greater amount (15% versus 5%) to your overall daily calorie expenditure versus that of your planned exercise.

One way a mother can accomplish her NEAT goals is by setting a daily step goal. A daily step goal can be easily obtainable, as daily steps add up (especially if a mother is being mindful about staying active throughout the day). Taking the stairs versus the elevator, parking farther away from a location, playing with your kids, walking the dog, etc., are all ways in which you can contribute toward your NEAT and overall TDEE (total daily energy expenditure). The daily step goal, just like our TDEE, can be thought of in terms of a daily or even weekly average to help make the goal more obtainable. For example, with a step goal of 8,000 steps per day, she can spread this goal over a week by subtracting her daily contributions from her weekly total of 56,000 steps. Therefore, she can decide whether she contributes more or less on some days, towards her overall goal. In total, depending on a mother's contribution to her NEAT, she will be able to make possibly greater contributions toward her overall calorie output and, therefore, fat loss. The ReShapeHER program incorporates these contributions and allows a mother to use NEAT as her secret weapon to further aid her in her body fat loss efforts.

The ReShapeHER program is based on some of the CDC recommendations for Physical Activity Guidelines for Americans, as they state that "adults 18-64 years of age should get at least 150 minutes a week of moderate intensity activity such as brisk walking and at least two days a week of activities that strengthen muscles."[33] In addition to these guidelines and my own principles for utilizing cardiovascular activities to successfully achieve a stellar body composition, the ReShapeHER program understands the secret behind NEAT activities when it comes to cardiovascular output. Therefore, in each tailored plan, NEAT is accounted for outside of the EAT portion of the cardiovascular part of this program (although in some cases it can replace a Mother's EAT movements) with a minimum step goal of 8,000 steps/day.

This step count is based on my own personal experience and also backed by studies published by the National Institute of Health. According to the NIH, "higher daily step counts were associated with lower mortality risk from all causes." They found that "compared with taking 4,000 steps per day, a number considered to be low for adults, taking 8,000 steps per day was associated with a 51% lower risk for all-cause mortality (or death from all causes)."[34] Of course, these studies didn't delineate EEE (planned exercise) from NEAT (unplanned exercise); however, they emphasize the benefits of having a daily step count in general.

Taking NEAT into consideration, making a conscious, daily effort to grow this 15% overall contribution toward one's daily TDEE can ultimately make a greater impact over time than their planned energy expenditure (EAT). If you combine this with your body's energy requirements and the amount of energy it requires to digest, absorb, and metabolize the food, you can see how much your EAT contribution of 5% can seem much more nominal as compared to the 95% contribution your body's energy requirements and NEAT combined, can allow you to achieve.

With these percentages, you can see why one could argue that their EAT is not as important when it comes to calorie expenditure, and why just staying active and eating a healthy diet can be the best contributors toward fat loss. This is partially true, but again, doesn't take the entire fitness picture into consideration. Planned exercise still has an important place in a solid fitness plan in terms of its "abilities to allow for muscle hypertrophy, contributions towards cardiovascular health, contribute towards calorie expenditure, etc. When combined with NEAT, a mother can make the most impact when it comes to her overall cardiovascular efforts with her fitness plan.

APPLYING CARDIO TO YOUR FITNESS SEASON WITH NEAT (NON-EXERCISE ACTIVITY THERMOGENESIS):

It is critical to remember that when you are working towards achieving your ideal body composition as a mother, cardiovascular exercise can help improve endurance, oxygen utilization efficiency, and cardiac respiratory function, but it doesn't help grow muscle tissue and build overall strength as does resistance training. Additionally, general cardiovascular activities do not reduce muscle development and contribute towards a mother achieving her body composition goals when it comes to her overall calorie output. The most important thing a mother needs to remember is that she consistently accomplishes her cardiovascular activities with one she enjoys so she will most likely reach her body composition goals.

"Off" Season

During a Mother's "off" season, as her focus will be on growing lean muscle tissue (and this is best done with adequate calories and resistance training), her planned cardiovascular activities may decrease. This is because she is in less of a need for a larger calorie output, as she isn't as focused as she would be in her "on" season, with reducing overall body fat. In this season, as a mother is focused on ensuring she has time for her resistance training in her planned EAT workouts, cardio usually takes a back seat. Therefore, she may reduce her planned cardio to the 15-minute minimum as suggested in the ReShapeHER program or replace this with her NEAT (Non-Exercise Activity Thermogenesis) movements (on days she has less time). Replacing her EAT with NEAT (in lieu of accomplishing them both in any given day), allows for her movements to contribute to her calorie output, however, knowing that this calorie contribution by doing this, won't amount to as much as doing them both in the same day. However, doing this will still allow for a mother to continue accomplishing her step targets suggested in this program (8000 steps/day).

In addition to a mother choosing to lower her cardiovascular movements in an "off" season to allow more time for resistance training, she may also do this to allow for more energy conservation for her to accomplish her lifts. By doing this, a mother can more successfully contribute the most amount of her energy to recruiting her muscle fibers in her lifts, in order to effectively build her lean muscle tissue during this season. Also, a mother might decide to accomplish her lifts via circuit training. With this type of training, a mother is able to incorporate endurance, cardiovascular and resistance training together, as she may rotate through various exercises in this program with less rest time or incorporate some HIIT (high-intensity training) exercises in between her lifts. The great thing is that the ReShapeHER program allows for a mother to make this individualized choice as to how she'd like to accomplish her cardiovascular movements according to her season. Also, the ReShapeHER program also supports a mother using her body composition data to determine her progress, so she can understand how successfully she's making progress with growing her lean muscle tissue during her "off" season

"On" Season

During a mother's "on" season, she can reach her goals within a short period of time by using the greatest secret weapon when it comes to achieving her body fat loss goals in the ReShapeHER program—her NEAT. **Considering a mother's NEAT will contribute 15% versus 5% towards her overall daily caloric output, she can use this to her advantage!** As a mother progresses through her "on" season, she can increase her overall daily caloric output by making sure she accomplishes BOTH her maximum EAT and NEAT recommendations in order to drive her calorie output as high as she can, increasing her body fat loss. When this is done in addition to her resistance training and a solid nutritional plan, she will start to see faster results that will lead her to her overall body composition goals.

In addition to a mother using NEAT, she may also choose to change her EAT from LISS (low-intensity, steady state) cardio to HIIT (high-intensity, interval training) cardiovascular movements to drive additional cardiovascular output. Or, she may choose to keep EAT at a lower intensity, as she may not have the energy reserves to do HIIT movements, and may choose to just increase her overall NEAT.

During an "on" season, it is critical to understand that our efforts that contribute to body fat loss are also what drive metabolic adaptation (this is why this season shouldn't last forever!) In order to continue contributing to body fat loss, a solid nutritional plan is required that readjusts one's TDEE (total daily energy expenditure) over time, as well as a solid fitness plan. The ReShapeHER program includes lifts that will continue to challenge a mother's muscle over time, in addition to suggested "Progressive Overload" practices (discussed in next chapter). Additionally, cardiovascular movements shouldn't remain the same in order to fight metabolic adaptations, as a mother would achieve her best results by alternating her favorite activities so her body can make even greater achievements towards her fat loss goals. For example, if she tends to do long walks for her NEAT activities, she may decide to do some alternating bike rides or light jogs for her EAT. A mother might choose to alternate a walk with a run some weeks. Regardless of what type of cardiovascular activities a mother chooses to do and at what intensities, it is important to understand that they should be changed over a period of time in order to prevent adaptations.

"Maintenance" Season

Because the goal of "maintenance" season for a mother is to keep her body at status quo, she has the opportunity to use her cardiovascular choices more freely during this time. Should she feel the need to increase her calorie output when she may have consumed too much or plans to, she can do more planned exercises, increase her NEAT, etc. Conversely, when she isn't trying to find the balance for this, she can enjoy her planned exercise and possibly replace them with NEAT depending on her circumstances. She has the ability to use both her EAT and NEAT to her advantage, depending on how well she knows her body and is able to maintain her current composition.

During the "maintenance" season, however, some mothers want to maintain some form of status quo but also grow their muscle while doing so. This is absolutely possible but not done as quickly as it would be in an "off" season. This can be accomplished by making resistance training a priority, although her calorie input won't be as high as "off" season, merely supporting her current TDEE and body composition (although it would still need to be recalculated and possibly adjusted due to her composition changes). It will be critical during a Mother's "maintenance" season, to ensure that she's continually evaluating her progress with body composition values instead of scale weight values to determine her possible muscle growth and/or status quo. This will ensure that she won't make a prejudgment when it comes to entering an "on" season "as it relates to weight gain from body fat", when in fact, she may when in fact, she may be growing her muscle or dealing with other phenomena (hormones, inflammation, etc.).

Calorie Tracking with Cardio

Movement tracking has grown in popularity within the fitness world, as the understanding of NEAT and its overall contribution toward one's TDEE has grown. The ReShapeHER program has been designed with this in mind, and recommends a wearable device to track daily steps in order for mothers to reach their fitness goals. These wearable devices are easy to find and have become part of the norm. According to CNET, the Pew Research Center reported in 2020 that "about one in five US adults regularly wears a smartwatch or fitness band." They state on their website that "we have more access than ever to data about our heart rate, how much sleep and activity we're getting and our overall well-being."[35] This is exciting news, especially for mothers who have little time and are always on the go, knowing they can make valuable contributions toward their NEAT that can be somewhat tracked.

Although our NEAT and EAT can be effectively tracked, there are still variabilities in their precision, as their numbers are often based on generalizations and as only as good as the technology allows them to be. Most of the calorie-tracking capabilities of cardio equipment in a local gym can often be inaccurate, leading someone to believe they are contributing to a greater expenditure than they are. The best way we can understand calorie output is through the generalizations we are provided. The best generalizations can only come from specific body composition tests, which can give you a more specific calorie expenditure for a specified period of time for each cardio activity specific to you. However, without this, the best way to understand what the calorie output values from cardio would be is through averages or "rules of thumb." For example, a "rule of thumb" is that you can burn about 100 calories per mile of walking for a 180-pound person and 65 calories per mile for a 120-pound person. Outside of these generalizations, what we are left with is our own individual results over time. This is why it's imperative that when doing a fitness plan you keep track of your progress to ensure that what you are doing is effective for you and your body specifically.

CARDIO—PUTTING IT ALL TOGETHER

Ultimately, solid fitness plans should be centered around long-term goals of building stronger bodies built for long-term health, not short, intermittent ones that are only focused on calorie output alone for body fat loss. The reason why we, as mothers, fall into the pitfalls of being "cardio bunnies" is because we can often be so motivated by immediacy and our short-term goals, forgetting the importance of how our long-term goals ultimately contribute to our general health and well-being. We are part of a society that is motivated by certain sizes and numbers, as if these are the true identifiers of health, when in reality these numbers don't reflect the condition of someone's health and longevity.

When it comes to a mother's overall TDEE contribution, the way that someone should view exercise is knowing that by incorporating daily, consistent energy expenditures, they are setting themselves up for long-term fitness success. Knowing that this long-term success is their primary goal, they will then think of their cardiovascular contributions less in terms of how it contributes to their TDEE but rather more on the importance it places on their long-term health. It is important to remember that although we become calorie-centric as we have a daily responsibility to stay within our TDEE without gaining weight, there are many ways we can make progress toward our daily calorie expenditures with our nutrition and overall movements versus being tied to a cardio machine. The ReShapeHER program isn't designed around short-term goals or efforts designed for body fat loss, solely focused on contributing toward energy expenditure, but rather long-term goals for health longevity. With our long-term goals in mind, we learn to appreciate exercise as a way to work toward optimal health no matter the type of contribution it makes toward our TDEE.

Practicing that both resistance training and cardio in a solid fitness plan, as well as maintaining an active lifestyle that contributes to your overall NEAT, are the keys to ensuring that you benefit from the best practices that will result in you having your best body composition. The ReShapeHER program allows a mother to accomplish this so she can reach her fitness goals **in as little as 4-6 weeks!**

CHAPTER 10 CLIFF NOTES

- Movement in general is an integral part of a solid fitness plan.
- The cardiovascular exercise portion of the ReShapeHER program is less important in terms of the type that is done, other than it is done consistently and it is something you enjoy.
- Although resistance training is necessary for the growth and development of muscle tissue, cardiovascular exercises contribute more to our caloric output than resistance training.
- Whether you choose to do HIIT (high-intensity interval training) or LIIS (low-intensity steady state) cardio, the same body fat loss goal can be accomplished.
- Oftentimes mothers tend to put their calorie deficit efforts into overdrive when they want to lose body fat. When combined with dieting too hard or long, especially if we do it too frequently we negate an optimal metabolism.
- Your NEAT—your Non-Exercise Activity Thermogenesis makes up 15% of your daily expenditure (as compared to your EAT—Exercise Activity Thermogenesis at 5%).
- One way a mother can accomplish her NEAT goals is by setting a daily step goal. This is why the ReShapeHER program includes a daily step goal for every mother at 8,000 steps per day
- Establishing your fitness goals around your fitness "seasons", allowing your body the proper amount of time to build lean muscle tissue, followed by a period of time to effectively lose body fat, is how you reach your body composition goals.
- Mothers can use their "cardiovascular activities (whether EAT or NEAT)" to their advantage in any of their seasons, whether it be "off" season, "on" season or "maintenance" season.

- NEAT and EAT can be effectively tracked, however, trackers often base their information on generalizations. This is why it's critical for mothers to understand and track their individual progress to cardiovascular exercises.
- Solid fitness plans should be centered around long-term goals of building stronger bodies built for long-term health, not short, intermittent ones that are only focused on calorie output alone for body fat loss.
- The ReShapeHER program isn't designed around short-term goals or efforts designed for body fat loss alone, solely focused on contributing toward energy expenditure, but rather focusing on having long-term goals that result in a better body composition.

NOTES

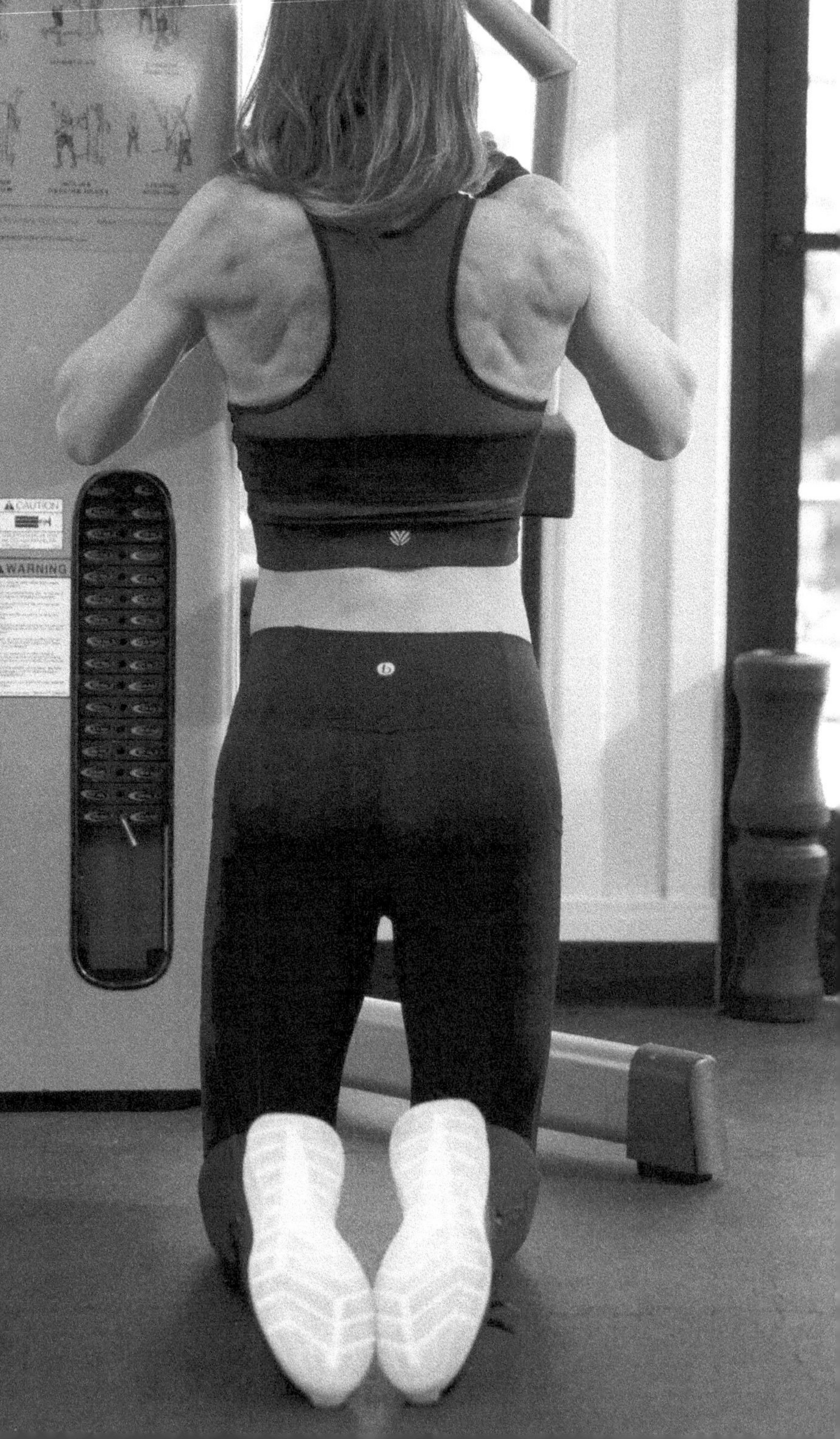
CAUTION
WARNING

11

Understanding Progressive Overload

I'VE DISCUSSED IN THE PREVIOUS chapter the importance of resistance training for mothers and how this is the key to developing a better body composition by growing your lean muscle tissue. This lean muscle tissue, along with a healthy body fat, will contribute to an aesthetically appealing body composition. The process of growing lean muscle tissue is done with a successful diet, as well as a resistance training program that incorporates a process called Progressive Overload. Progressive Overload is when you gradually increase the weight ("load"), frequency, or number of repetitions in your strength training routine. This practice allows you to challenge your body over time, driving your musculoskeletal system to get stronger ("hypertrophy") by increasing the tension on your muscles over a given period of time and ultimately leading to muscle growth over time.

Progressive Overload can be done with both resistance training and also with cardiovascular exercises (the ReShapeHER program includes guideline information for resistance training only). This process is done in order to prevent plateaus (when your body adapts to a particular training stimulus that it is under and no longer responds). It is important, however, to understand how to practice Progressive Overload correctly and the many ways you can provide your musculoskeletal system a challenge, and at the same time, prevent injury in doing so.

The ReShapeHER program allows a mother to use it successfully in order to build a lean and toned physique over time.

Gauging Personal Exertion

When it comes to resistance training, understanding how to gauge one's personal exertion abilities becomes critical in knowing not only how to begin a resistance training program, but also how to progress from that point. It is imperative to know at what point it is critical to start adding more weight to your muscle ("load") that was once your maximum capacity for a particular muscle group. You have to efficiently ask yourself if you're working to full capacity on a particular muscle group, using the mind-muscle connection, and keeping track of the progress you're making over time if you want to make serious changes to your body composition. Before initiating the practice of Progressive Overload, it is critical that a mother consistently does the same lifts over time in order to ensure that she is ready to apply more "load" (weight) through these movements. The more tracking you do in this area, especially in the beginning, the more fluent you become.

There are many fitness influencers who will often promote a continual variation of lifts that don't follow Progressive Overload practices. These influencers do this to attract followers, as their constant introductions of new movements keep things new and interesting. However, these constant lift variations don't allow for a mother to challenge specific muscle groups to capacity over time, and in turn, they don't strengthen as much as they could if they were to apply the principles of Progressive Overload. Although the same, consistent lifts aren't always exciting to promote, they do result in progress. Therefore, with a tried and true fitness plan that includes solid resistance training lifts, coupled with the principles of Progressive Overload applied over time, a better body composition can be expected with a greater muscle development.

Progressive Overload happens faster the more you push toward your failure mark for exertion, meaning you are lifting toward maximum amounts of weight for each set, for each muscle group being exercised.

However, pushing toward failure shouldn't be the goal for every workout, as the muscle needs adequate rest over time, in order to allow for growth and also to prevent injury. It is also not a perfect science, and as with weight loss, results are not produced in a linear fashion.

The ReShapeHER Conservative Approach

There are many things to consider when we talk about Progressive Overload—the exhaustion that occurs when you push toward a maximum weight with a specific muscle group, the nutrition required to fuel this, the rest that is needed to support growth, the time designated to this practice between each working muscle group, and also practicing this all while avoiding injury in the process. These are the reasons why Progressive Overload should be done in a conservative manner, starting low and going slow in order to successfully achieve your goals, especially when starting a new fitness plan.

Additionally, increasing muscular resistance ("load") shouldn't be the goal for every workout, which is why the ReShapeHER program recommends doing this once every 2-4 weeks, allowing for different muscle groups to adjust to heavier weights over time. This in turn also helps to prevent the practice of "pushing to failure" with every workout, as the muscle groups adjust to their new load weights over this period of time. Regardless of the fitness advancements made or tenure of a mother practicing Progressive Overload, the ReShapeHER program recommends a conservative approach to this technique, encouraging her to have proper form as she increases her weight for each lift yet also prevents injury.

ACSM Recommendations for Gauging Effort with Progressive Overload

According to the American College of Sports Medicine (ACSM) guidelines, in their website brochure for Resistance Training for Health and Fitness, they recommend the maximum load for the four category types of resistance training: Muscular Strength, Muscular Power, Muscular Endurance, and Muscular Hypertrophy/Definition. The ReShapeHER

Program focuses on the Muscular Hypertrophy/Definition category, as this is the one that most mothers would fall into—that is, they want to quickly make changes to their body composition.

The ACSM recommends a "load of 70-85% 1RPM (1 rep maximum) for novice to intermediate, 70-100% 1RPM for advanced."[36] This means that when a mother starts out as a beginner, she would be lifting a load weight of 70-85% (the percentage of effort you would give to a weight that in one repetition would require your maximum effort for a particular muscle group you are exercising). For example, when doing a bicep curl, if I was using a 40-pound barbell or two 20-pound dumbbells on each side, I would be within a 70-85% 1RPM if I felt like this weight was heavy enough to engage my muscles and challenge me to about 70-85% of my effort in lifting it, to complete my number of sets/reps I intended to do. Without getting too technical, this means a mother would be pushing close to failure but NOT at failure. She would stay at this maximum effort of 70-85% 1RPM until over time she felt like her effort wasn't as high, and then she would increase the weight slowly, practicing the art of Progressive Overload.

So you can see, the standard way of practicing Progressive Overload can simply be done by gauging effort. This process becomes very individualized and also varies over time as compared from one individual to the next. When it becomes time to increase the weight (or "load"), this should be done in a very conservative manner and the new weight ("load") should also be gauged by this same amount of effort or 1RPM.

Most gyms offer lower weight counts of two or five pounds to allow for you to practice Progressive Overload over time. The importance of documentation is critical once you start the process, not only to remember your new starting weight and how you're progressing, but also to prevent injury from lifting a weight that falls outside of your 70-85% 1RPM range. With continual practice, this art becomes easier over time. In my experience, most advanced lifters and experienced bodybuilders will tell you that you need to allow yourself at least 2-4 weeks before advancing to a new heavier weight to ensure that you are truly executing the exercise correctly and in good form before moving to a higher weight.

The ACSM recommends that in order to reduce the risk of over training, "a dramatic increase in volume should be avoided." They recommend that a "2-10% increase in the load should be applied only when the individual can comfortably perform the current workload for 1-2 repetitions over the desired number on two consecutive training sessions."[37] For example, this would mean that if you took the same example above for the bicep curl of 40 pounds at a 70-85% of 1RPM over three sets of 12 repetitions, let's say, you would be able to comfortably do about three sets of 12 repetitions for about 2-3 training sessions for that particular muscle group with the ReShapeHER program (within the recommended 2-4 weeks), before you would move the weight to a higher one like 45 pounds.

Ways to Drive Progressive Overload

There are a few other ways to drive Progressive Overload to the musculoskeletal system that aren't talked about as much as adjusting weight over time. Progressive Overload can also be accomplished through other ways such as: increasing your reps over time, increasing how often you train, changing the tempo of your movement, increasing your range of motion, and decreasing your rest time between sets (with a few other ways not mentioned).

When you increase your reps over time, you can still progress by staying within the recommended rep range for your goal but by adding maybe 1-2 additional reps in that range in order to make it more challenging. For example, if you were doing 12 repetitions of leg presses, you could increase that to 15 and still stay within the Muscular Definition range and allow for a greater challenge to fuel Progressive Overload. You might decide to switch from the ReShapeHER program's 3-Day Fitness Plan to the 5-Day Fitness Plan (discussed in the next chapter) in order to train additional days to allow for greater Muscular Definition and support this technique.

You can also change the tempo of your movements when executing them. For example, if doing hip thrusts, you can execute this by doing them at a faster speed or doing one full thrust, followed by a half thrust, followed by a full thrust, and repeating this. You can increase your range of motion to drive Progressive Overload by doing things such as deeper squats to allow for greater muscle recruitment. Additionally, you can decrease your rest time between sets by allowing for a one-minute rest time versus two-minute, or you can perform supersets (two exercises that are performed back-to-back), often followed by a short rest. *Personally, supersets have been my secret weapon, especially when performing them for isolation exercises for the glutes. They allow me to effectively double the amount of work I am doing while keeping the recovery period the same as they are when you complete individual exercises. Supersets are a great way, if you can, to maximize the time allotment you may have in the gym with a busy schedule!*

Progressive Overload, by way of increasing how often you train over time, can also be accomplished by a mother who decides to switch from the ReShapeHER 3-Day Fitness Plan to the 5-Day Fitness Plan. When a mother decides that she will be designating more time to her fitness routine, this allows her to resistance train more hours of the week, therefore contributing to more time under tension for her muscle groups. By way of Progressive Overload, this "time under tension" will lead her to having more significant muscle strength/growth over time should she choose to exercise the 5-Day Fitness Plan versus the 3-Day Fitness Plan.

One of the ways a mother can apply Progressive Overload to her lifts is by using a "circuit training" approach. In this type of training, she will raise her heart rate by performing a consecutive series of timed exercises, one after the other with varying amounts of rest between each exercise. Examples of these types of exercises would be push-ups, sit-ups, squats, lunges, etc. This can be a great option for mothers that want to burn more calories in less time. With this style of programming, it's important for a beginner to start out with lighter "loads" than her current load, to safely accommodate for the increased intensity until she feels comfortable at a heavier load to accomplish the lifts in the given time. Additionally, it is critical for a mother to perform the movements that require a higher level of exertion first in her planned workout.

When to Apply Progressive Overload

When it comes to the period of time in which you can apply changes to your workouts by way of Progressive Overload, the National Academy of Sports Medicine (NASM) discusses the principles of Progressive Overload in its article *Progressive Overload Explained: Grow Muscle & Strength Today*. "The Principle of Progression states that increases in time, weight or intensity should be kept within 10% or less each week to allow for a gradual adaptation while minimizing risk of injury. Without this progressive overloading, muscle growth will plateau."[38] This article goes on to say under the section *When Should You Progressively Overload?* that "each client's needs will vary based on training regimens, genetics, nutrition and many other factors. It is also dependent upon the client's goals (i.e. weight loss versus increasing muscle). The most common periodization would schedule in progressions every 2-4 weeks." Therefore, this article suggests that after someone can successfully lift a weight with good form, they can advance at no more than 10% or less of an increase to their load each week, with this being scheduled on average every 2-4 weeks. However, the article does state that "there are times when client needs may call for Progressive Overloading weekly or within a single workout."[39]

Therefore, Progressive Overloading is very individualized, and because of this, special attention must be paid to the ability of each individual to lift their goal weight successfully and with great form before advancing by way of Progressive Overload. The ReShapeHER understands the principles of Progressive Overload and incorporates these principles into its 3-Day and 5-Day Fitness Plans discussed in the following chapter, as recommended by the NASM at *no more than <10% every 2-4 weeks.*

As with weight loss, Progressive Overload isn't accomplished in a linear fashion. An "on" season may result in a reduction in scale weight right away. However, the last 10 or so pounds can often feel like they take much longer. Progressive Overload can be similar. In the beginning, Progressive Overload can be much easier as you advance through weight loads quickly, but as they get heavier over time, it can often take months to make any advancements. Additionally, when you are in a calorie deficit, you may not make as much progress as you do when you're maintaining your TDEE or in a calorie surplus. This is because you have less available energy to put toward your heavier lifts, therefore resulting in less progress. However, it is still possible to achieve your goals regardless of the season you're in. By applying the principles of Progressive Overload, if you have taken some time away from resistance training (with injury, illness, vacation, etc), you can return to the strength levels you were once at n due time as you practice it.

"No Pain No Gain" Doesn't Apply

This concept of Progressive Overload can often be misconstrued when it comes to overall weight ("load"). The term "Overload" can be thought of as though we are just piling on weight that the muscle is forced to lift in order to create growth. This is not the case. In fact, what we are doing when we practice the art of Progressive Overload is allowing the muscle groups we are targeting to continue to break down, and in turn, recruit more fibers to be able to lift the same weight we have been using to grow them week over week. It is only at this point of muscle recruitment and growth that we add more weight (or "load") to these muscles as we recognize that they are capable of lifting it due to their growth. Thinking of Progressive Overload in this manner helps to avoid injury and allows for a conservative and successful approach to resistance training over time.

This misconstrued concept of Progressive Overload is what often promotes the idea of the "No Pain, No Gain" mentality when it comes to lifting. It encourages the idea that muscle soreness and pain is a requirement to make substantial muscle growth. This is certainly not the case and can often discourage many people (especially women) from wanting to practice resistance training in the first place. Although acute muscle soreness can be experienced during or shortly after a workout, and DOMS (delayed muscle soreness) can be experienced normally a day or two after a workout, both aren't required in order to have a productive workout that provides you successful results.

Oftentimes DOMS specifically is a result of starting a new exercise routine or simply challenging muscle groups that aren't normally challenged, if you're not a beginner. It is important to understand that it is not a requirement in order to know that you're working out hard enough or that you may be missing out on fitness gains if you don't experience it.

Personally, I avoid muscle soreness by practicing my Progressive Overload efforts more conservatively while still continuing to make advancements. I've suffered from bad cases of DOMS that have set me back many days in order to recover, and for me and my busy lifestyle, it's not worth it. I'm sure many mothers would feel this way as they probably don't have the time to nurse themselves back to health in addition to their kids. If you experience this, you may have to take a day off from training and rest, take a few cold or hot baths, take a topical analgesic, get a massage, or use an anti-inflammatory medication. Regardless of how you choose to relieve it, time is usually the only treatment, and continual movement is important to ease pain and stiffness in the joints.

The Downside of Resistance Bands

When it comes to Progressive Overload and weight ("load") on the muscle, this is the area where resistance bands alone can become a problem for the more advanced lifter who is working out at home. Resistance bands are a wonderful way to start a resistance training program; however, they have their limitations. They only allow for a certain amount of resistance ("load") for a particular muscle group. Once a muscle group has grown and hypertrophy has been experienced that creates a lower effort for the lifter, they don't allow for a maximum amount of hypertrophy when used alone.

Resistance bands can be doubled up; however, the same can happen even with the resistance of two or more bands. When this occurs, a lifter falls into a load category that ACSM defines as "Muscular Endurance."[40] This is when a muscle or muscle group repeatedly exerts a sub-maximal resistance (by their definition, "a load lower than 70% of 1RM"). Therefore, the muscle can possibly be maintained through the continual resistance and nutritious diet to support the efforts. However, it won't be in an environment that allows for muscular hypertrophy (growth) due to the decline in load effort.

It is at this point that someone using resistance bands alone for their resistance-training workouts may decide to purchase weights to add to their home gym, get a gym membership to give them access to heavier weights, or continue to practice the art of training for Muscular Endurance. However, for a more advanced lifter, resistance bands can be used as an adjunct to weights to allow for a means of accomplishing progressive overload, if used correctly.

ACSM Recommendations for Lift Frequencies

Whether or not you use weights or resistance bands, the frequency at which you practice your lifting efforts also depends on how you advance with Progressive Overload. The ACSM recommends that for all four of the Muscular groups mentioned, novice individuals should train the entire body 2-3 days per week. Intermediate individuals should train three days if using a total-body workout or four days if using an upper/lower body split routine (each muscle group 2x/week). Advanced lifters can train 4-6 days per week, training each major muscle group 1-2 times per week. Elite weightlifters and bodybuilders may benefit from using very high frequencies, such as two workouts per day for

4-5 days per week.[41] The ReShapeHER program has taken the ACSM recommendations into consideration with both the 3-Day and 5-Day Fitness Plans that allow for a any mother, from a novice to advanced weightlifter, to achieve her best body composition.

PEDS (Performance Enhancing Drugs)

Performance Enhancing Drugs are becoming more popular not only in the fitness world, but also in the general public, as more people are learning about and obtaining access to them. They have the ability or potential to drastically alter the human body and biological functions by increasing muscle, athletic performance, etc. There are many risks associated with these drugs that I won't discuss in this book. However, I include this section on them, as it is important for a mother to know that she can achieve an incredibly toned body composition without them. By adopting solid fitness and nutritional practices like the ones in the ReShapeHER program, and applying the principles of Progressive Overload, any mother (regardless of their starting point), can achieve a better body composition and athletic performance with consistency over time.

This ReShapeHER program ensures that each muscle group is being hit successfully each week, whether you are a beginner or at a more advanced fitness level with both the 3-Day and 5-Day Fitness Plans that are discussed in the next chapter. It takes Progressive Overload into consideration, allowing for successful muscle growth in order for a mother to obtain a great body composition, as well as maintain her Muscular Endurance!

PROGRESSIVE OVERLOAD – PUTTING IT ALL TOGETHER

Realistic fitness goals depend on how solid your fitness program is, how disciplined you are as a mother, what equipment you plan to work with, and what effort you plan to put forth in a resistance training program. For example, if your goal is to gain muscular tone but you only have access to bands at home and you're a beginner, you will be able to see some gains until you reach a point that you'll have to decide if the progress you've made is enough to continue doing what you're doing at home or you need to purchase weights or a gym membership (considering you are consistently practicing your resistance training at a recommended frequency and would like to reach your goals). Let's say you have a gym membership but you can only go three days a week but would like to achieve a better body composition. You'll need to ensure that you are practicing a resistance training program that allows for Progressive Overload and maximizes efforts for all of your muscle groups you'd like to target. The beauty of the ReShapeHER program is that this part has been thought out for you! In the following chapters, I discuss my recommended 3-Day and 5-Day Fitness Plans, which take all of this into consideration!

When it comes to Progressive Overload, a mother can successfully practice it with the ReShapeHER program. Both the 3-Day and 5-Day Fitness Plans allow for a busy mom to challenge each of her muscle groups at least once per week, allowing for her to implement the practice of Progressive Overload during a recommended 2-4 weeks at more than <10% during this time, as she advances with her fitness. Additionally, whether a mother is working out at home or in the gym, her Progressive Overload goals can be achieved. The ReShapeHER program takes any mother's fitness levels, time allowances, and Progressive Overload concepts into consideration, helping her achieve her fitness goals in a short period of time!

CHAPTER 11 CLIFF NOTES

- Progressive Overload is when you gradually increase the weight ("load"), frequency, or number of repetitions in your strength training routine. This practice allows you to challenge your body over time, driving your musculoskeletal system to get stronger ("hypertrophy") by increasing the tension on your muscles over a given period of time and ultimately leading to muscle growth.
- The ACSM Progressive Overload recommendation is for a maximum effort of 70-85% 1RPM for beginners and 70-100% for advanced lifters and is incorporated in the ReShapeHER program.
- Progressive Overload can also be accomplished through other ways such as: increasing your reps over time, increasing how often you train, changing the tempo of your movement, increasing your range of motion, and decreasing your rest time between sets, etc. Supersets can also be a secret weapon to drive Progressive Overload!
- The ReShapeHER program follows the recommended NASM periodization recommendations for Progressive Overload at no more than <10% every 2-4 weeks.
- Progress with Progressive Overload doesn't happen in a linear fashion.
- By applying the principles of Progressive Overload, if you have taken some time away from resistance training (with injury, illness, vacation, etc), you can return to the strength levels you were once at over time.
- Progressive Overload shouldn't be practiced with a "No Pain, No Gain" mentality. Experiencing DOMS doesn't dictate successful resistance training.
- The downside of resistance bands is that they only allow for a

certain amount of resistance ("load") for a particular muscle group and experienced lifters will progress beyond this when the principles of Progressive Overload are applied.

- This ReShapeHER program ensures that each muscle group is being met by the ACSM recommendations for resistance training frequencies, whether you are a beginner or at a more advanced fitness level with both the 3-Day and 5-Day Fitness Plans.
- When it comes to Progressive Overload, a mother can successfully practice it with the ReShapeHER program. Both the 3-Day and 5-Day Fitness Plans allow for a busy Mom to challenge each of her muscle groups at least once per week, allowing for her to implement the practice of Progressive Overload during a recommended 2-4 weeks at a conservative <10%, as she advances with her fitness journey.

NOTES

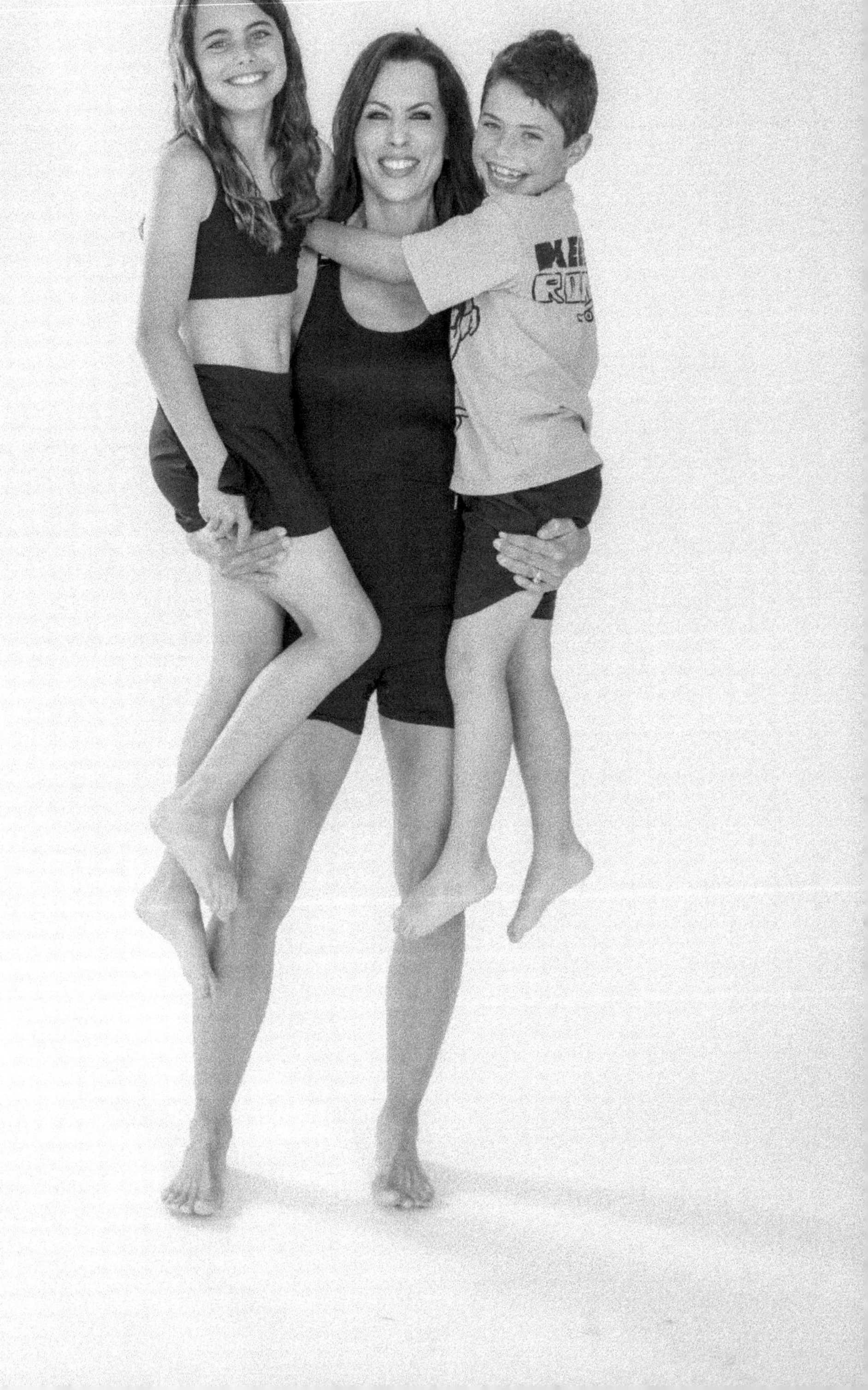

12

The ReShapeHER 3-Day and 5-Day Fitness Plans

IN THIS CHAPTER, YOU WILL be able to apply all of the information you've learned in this book when it comes to your nutrition and fitness goals, and practice it with one of two versions of the ReShapeHER program with the 3-Day Fitness Plan or the 5-Day Fitness Plan. Both of these plans can be tailored to any mother regardless of her lifestyle, where she chooses to practice them and are very easy to follow. Both of these plans have resulted in my own personal fitness success and the reason why I've been able to obtain my optimal body composition after having two kids. I was also able to achieve this in my 40s and become a bodybuilding competitor! The 3-Day and 5-Day Fitness Plans have also resulted in the success of the many mothers who have practiced them in my pilot programs. So, ladies, read on as you decide which plan works best for your lifestyle and be ready to achieve some great results **in as little as 4-6 weeks!**

RESISTANCE TRAINING FREQUENCY

The Resistance Training part of the ReShapeHER program incorporates not only specific lifts that have been instrumental in my own personal success as a mother, but it also incorporates scientific principles from the National Strength and Conditioning Association. The ReShape-HER program follows the NSCA in providing guidelines for novice or intermediate training to be three sessions per week and advanced at 4-6 sessions per week for individuals to maintain strength and experience gains,[42] which also suffice the requirements for strength training recommended by the Center for Disease Control[43] as well as the American Heart Association.[44] For these reasons, the resistance training portion of the 3-Day Fitness Plan recommends a minimum of three days of resistance training, as well as an advanced level of 5 days of resistance training per week (incorporating both Compound and Isolation lifts) in the 5-Day Fitness Plan, dedicated to non-consecutive days of training the specific muscle groups mentioned.

Sets and Reps

The Fit Moms 3-Day and 5-Day Fitness Plans incorporate the ACE guidelines for sets and reps, suggesting a beginning goal for a woman at 1-2 sets for each lift at a range of 8-15 reps. As she progresses, the suggestion is that a woman performs each lift at 3-4 sets of a rep range and 8-15 thereafter. Additionally, when she practices the method of Progressive Overload, in order to prevent injury, she may choose to lower her set and/or rep range to accommodate for the increase in weight until she reaches her maximum suggested sets of 3-4 and rep range of 8-15.

Progressive Overload applications

Taking Progressive Overload into consideration, the suggested lifts in the ReShapeHER Program shouldn't be changed (in terms of their weight/"load") prior to every 2-4 weeks, to ensure that proper muscle strength and form has been accomplished when doing them. *Remember, the general recommendation for Progressive Overload is given: an increase in load at no more than <10% every 2-4 weeks. (Note: With the 3-Day Fitness Plan, because each muscle group isn't being worked as frequently, adjustments should not be made as soon, especially when being compared to the 5-Day Fitness Plan.)*

NEAT (Non-Exercise Activity Thermogenesis)

NEAT is listed every day, as this should be accomplished as an addition to a mother's EE (planned exercise) and diet, contributing to her overall 8K step count goal. NEAT can be accomplished with activities such as additional walking, chasing after kids, cleaning, running errands, etc. All of a Mother's cardiovascular activities (EE and NEAT) can all be calculated using a recommended step counter of choice. NEAT activities can be counted towards a Mother's planned exercise (EE), should a mother not have time to accomplish a planned exercise for that day. There is no set time for NEAT as with planned exercise. *Remember, it can be used as a secret weapon for additional calorie output when a woman is trying to increase her energy expenditure (especially in an "on" season), as an addition to her planned exercise.*

Time Commitment for EAT (Exercise Activity Thermogenesis—"planned" exercise)

When it comes to an overall fitness time commitment for the 3-Day and 5-Day Fitness Plan, a minimum of 15 minutes should be a goal for each day, (not to exceed 2 hours). This should include all time allotted for any planned exercise (resistance or cardio), and also include any time allotted for warm-ups, cool-downs, etc.

CHOOSING A PLAN

The 3-Day Fitness Plan is designed for a mother who is beginning her fitness journey or for one who has a limited amount of time to dedicate to her fitness plan. The 5-Day Fitness Plan is designed for a mother who is able to contribute at least five total days each week to her fitness plan. She is either moving past the 3-Day Fitness Plan or has previous fitness experience that allows her to take on this plan successfully. With the successful execution of these plans as well as combining them with the recommended ReShapeHER nutritional guidelines, any mother should be able to achieve the body composition she desires.

As a beginner, allowing yourself time for your body to adapt to a new program is imperative. Although in the long run I recommend practicing the 5-Day Fitness Plan for ultimate results, a beginner would need to allow for more rest time to build up to this weekly consistency, and sometimes our schedules don't always allow for a five-day-a-week contribution. Nonetheless, the 3-Day Fitness Plan will still allow for fantastic results if followed with consistency. If you're a beginner, I would recommend doing the 3-Day Fitness Plan until you've built yourself up to accommodate the 5-Day Fitness Plan.

One of the most common occurrences that happens with a new program is the development of inflammation and soreness as a result of introducing your body to new movements. It is critical to allow your body time to rest and recover from this temporary inflammatory state, which may include fatigue, DOMS (delayed-onset muscle soreness), water weight gain, etc. As a beginner, you must listen to your body and advance only when you have recovered from the onset of inflammation and have developed a nice base of muscle strength. This fitness portion of the plan (when combined with the nutritional outline) will ensure that you are getting the best results possible during this time, even with greater periods of rest.

One of the biggest differences between this 3-Day Fitness Plan and the 5-Day Fitness Plan is the amount of rest time that is dedicated to each muscle group in terms of resistance training. This rest time is incorporated in order to avoid inflammation and to allow for proper muscle growth. LISS (low-intensity, steady-state) cardiovascular activities are also recommended for the 3-Day Fitness Plan for beginners. As a mother advances through the 3-Day Fitness Plan, she can decide at what point her body can accommodate possible HIIT (high-intensity, interval training), but it is not required for either plan.

ReShapeHER 3-Day Fitness Plan

The ReShapeHER program's 3-Day Fitness Plan is a great starting point for a beginner or for a mother who doesn't have as much time during the week to dedicate to her fitness. This plan can be accomplished at home or in a gym and can be easily tailored to fit any type of lifestyle or fitness goal. Regardless of the additional rest time the 3-Day Fitness Plan incorporates versus the 5-Day Fitness Plan, a mother can stay in this plan over a lifetime and experience amazing results regardless of what season she's in.

Time Commitment Per Week

Minimum: Three 15 min. sessions of Resistance training per week, three 15 min sessions of cardio per week (can be traded for NEAT when needed), seven days of 8,000 steps of movement per week (totaling 56,000 steps that can be spread throughout the week), and 20 min total full-body stretching.

Average: Three 30 min. sessions of Resistance training per week, three 30 min sessions of cardio per week (can be traded for NEAT when needed), seven days of 8,000 steps of movement per week (totaling 56,000 steps that can be spread throughout the week)

Advanced: Three 60 min. sessions (1 optional) of Resistance training per week (taking advantage of "optional" sessions), four 60 min. sessions of cardio (can be traded for NEAT when needed), seven days of 8,000 steps of movement per week (totaling 56,000 steps that can be spread throughout the week), and 20 min full-body stretching.

EAT (Planned Exercise—Resistance Training and Cardio)

For resistance training, the ReShapeHER 3-Day Fitness Plan allows for muscle group(s) to be exercised at least once per week. For each planned workout, 50% time contribution will be spent towards resistance training for days that it is programmed. (For example, for a 1 hour workout, at least 30 minutes would be paid to resistance training). Resistance training should include a 50/50 split of Compound and Isolation exercises for muscle groups listed equaling eight total lifts per muscle group(s) for that day, (with Compound lifts being the priority as they require more muscle engagement and should be done first and also prioritized over Isolation ones). For example, on Day 1 for Abs/Glutes, that would total a maximum of four total lifts for Abdominals (2 Compound and 2 Isolation) and four lifts for Glutes (2 Compound and 2 Isolation). *Day 5 is the only day that has three muscle groups, which would make the Compound lift total less than two per muscle group, as three muscle groups are being considered versus two.* Not every planned session will include all the lifts in either the Compound or Isolation categories, therefore, the lifts can be rotated throughout consecutive sessions. What this means with the 3-Day Fitness Plan, is that all of the Compound and Isolation lifts for a particular muscle group would be accomplished after 2 weeks with this plan. The ReShapeHER program recommends a minimum of 15 minutes of resistance training to a maximum of 60 minutes per planned session.

Resistance Training Equipment Needed

Gym Membership or Home Equipment listed below:

ReShapeHER Program Home Equipment Needs
Dumbbells
Medicine Ball or Heavy Duffle Bag
Resistance Bands - looped and open
Sturdy Chair/Table
Hanging Bar (or playground equipment)
Floor mat

Progressive Overload is included with the ReShapeHER program, as it recommends practicing it no more than <10% every 2-4 weeks (70-85% RPM for beginner, 70-100% for advanced). A mother can choose to maximize this practice, should she want to grow her lean muscle tissue to a greater degree depending on her season.

Planned cardiovascular exercises are programmed 5x/week in this plan (one day being optional), with two rest days built in. These exercises will be done second to resistance training for days where both are scheduled. Cardiovascular exercises should include the ones that a mother enjoys and one type isn't preferred over another. LISS (low-intensity, steady state) cardio is recommended for beginners who start with this plan. The ReShapeHER program recommends a minimum of 15 minutes of cardiovascular exercises to a maximum of 60 minutes per planned session.

NEAT (unplanned exercise)

The ReShapeHER program recommends a step tracker for these unplanned movements a mother can achieve just by having an active lifestyle. They should be counted separately from their EAT, however, on days that a mother may not have time to complete her EAT, she can replace them with her NEAT activities (knowing this will decrease her caloric output potential). This program also includes a minimum daily step count of 8,000 steps (even on rest days).

Cardio Requirements

Step counter/tracker for NEAT and EAT

Stretching Requirements

Floor mats

Nutrition

The ReShapeHER program recommends a mother use the calculator to determine her TDEE (based on her individual values), to understand the amount of calories and macronutrients she needs to consume, depending on her season. This TDEE should be recalculated, and possibly adjusted every 2-4 weeks based on a mother's weight and activity levels.

RESHAPEHER 3-DAY OUTLINE

Fitness Portion:

Day 1	Abs/Glutes + LISS (low-intensity, steady-state) Cardio + NEAT
Day 2	REST + NEAT + Flexibility
Day 3	Thighs/Hamstrings + LISS cardio + NEAT
Day 4	LISS cardio (optional) + NEAT
Day 5	Shoulders/Arms/Back + LISS cardio + NEAT
Day 6	LISS cardio + NEAT
Day 7	REST + NEAT + Flexibility

RESISTANCE TRAINING (EAT): 15 minutes minimum on recommended days; maximum 60 minutes (50% time contribution of total workout). Lifts are split 50/50 by choosing half compound and half isolation for each given muscle group (8 lifts maximum).

Progressive overload: no more than <10% every 2-4 weeks (70-85% RPM for beginner, 70-100% for advanced)

CARDIO (EAT): 15 minutes minimum on recommended days; should follow resistance training when combined with it; maximum 60 min.

LISS (low-intensity, steady-state recommended for 3-Day Fitness Plan as a beginner) can be replaced with NEAT

NEAT: Accomplished as an addition to EAT in order to reach daily minimum step goal of 8,000.

FLEXIBILITY: 20 minutes full-body stretching requirements per week

REST DAY: No planned Resistance Training or Cardio; includes NEAT goal of 8000 steps.

NUTRITION: TDEE based on season and followed, recalculated and possibly adjusted every 2-4 weeks depending on weight and/or activity levels.

ReShapeHER 3-Day Fitness Plan | Week 1

	RESISTANCE TRAINING AREA OF FOCUS	RESISTANCE TRAINING LIFTS (15-60 MINUTES)	CARDIO	NEAT	PROGRESSIVE OVERLOAD	FLEXIBILITY
MONDAY	Abs/Glutes	Back Squats, Sumo Deadlift, Hip Thrusts, Cable kick-back, Suitcase Deadlift, Medicine Ball slams, Abdominal Crunches, Hanging Knee Raise/ Twist, (max 8)	15-60 minutes (ex: Bike ride)	8000 steps	no more than <10% every 4 weeks (70-85% RPM for beginner, 70-100% for advanced)	X
TUESDAY	X	X	X	8000 steps	X	10 minutes of full body stretching
WEDNES-DAY	Thighs/ Hamstrings	Romanian Deadlift, Alternating Weighted step-ups, walking lunges, Leg press, seated/lying leg curls, cable side leg raises, cable pull-throughs, monster band walks (max 8)	15-60 minutes (ex: jog)	8000 steps	X	X
THURSDAY	X	X	X (optional)	8000 steps	X	X
FRIDAY	Shoulders/ Arms/ Back	Overhead Press, Single-arm front raise, pull-ups and chin-ups, barbell curls, single-arm dumbbell curls, bent-over barbell row, V-grip lat pulldown and single-arm seated cable row (max 8)	15-60 minutes (ex: planned walk)	8000 steps	X	X
SATURDAY	X	X	15-60 minutes (ex: row)	8000 steps	X	X
SUNDAY	X	X	X	8000 steps	X	10 minutes of full body stretching

ReShapeHER 3-Day Fitness Plan | Week 2						
	RESISTANCE TRAINING AREA OF FOCUS	RESISTANCE TRAINING LIFTS (15-60 MINUTES)	CARDIO	NEAT	PROGRESSIVE OVERLOAD	FLEXIBILITY
MONDAY	Abs/Glutes	Bulgarian Split Squats, Weighted Step-ups, Hip Abduction/ Adduction, Reverse Glute hyper, Bear Crawl, Single-leg Deadift, Seated Russian twist, Cable Ab pulldown (max 8)	15-60 minutes (ex: Bike ride)	8000 steps	no more than <10% every 4 weeks (70-85% RPM for beginner, 70-100% for advanced)	X
TUESDAY	X	X	X	8000 steps	X	10 minutes of full body stretching
WEDNES-DAY	Thighs/ Hamstrings	Romanian Deadlift, Alternating Weighted step-ups, walking lunges, Leg press, seated/lying leg curls, cable side leg raises, cable pull-throughs, monster band walks (max 8)	15-60 minutes (ex: swim)	8000 steps	X	X
THURSDAY	X	X	X (optional)	8000 steps	X	X
FRIDAY	Shoulders/ Arms/ Back	Push-ups, single-arm lateral raise, cable press-downs, kettlebell swings, single-arm tricep push-downs, inverted row, single-arm seated cable row, single-arm lat pulldown and straight-arm cable pulldown (max 8)	15-60 minutes (ex: ellipti-cal machine)	8000 steps	X	X
SATURDAY	X	X	15-60 minutes (ex: hiking)	8000 steps	X	X
SUNDAY	X	X	X	8000 steps	X	10 minutes of full body stretching

ReShapeHER 3-Day Fitness Plan | Week 3						
	RESISTANCE TRAINING AREA OF FOCUS	**RESISTANCE TRAINING LIFTS (15-60 MINUTES)**	**CARDIO**	**NEAT**	**PROGRESSIVE OVERLOAD**	**FLEXIBILITY**
MONDAY	Abs/Glutes	Back Squats, Sumo Deadlift, Hip Thrusts, Cable kick-back, Suitcase Deadlift, Medicine Ball slams, Abdominal Crunches, Hanging Knee Raise/ Twist, (max 8)	15-60 minutes (ex: pilates)	8000 steps	no more than <10% every 4 weeks (70-85% RPM for beginner, 70-100% for advanced)	X
TUESDAY	X	X	X	8000 steps	X	10 minutes of full body stretching
WEDNES-DAY	Thighs/ Hamstrings	Romanian Deadlift, Alternating Weighted step-ups, walking lunges, Leg press, seated/lying leg curls, cable side leg raises, cable pull-throughs, monster band walks (max 8)	15-60 minutes (ex: yoga)	8000 steps	X	X
THURSDAY	X	X	X (optional)	8000 steps	X	X
FRIDAY	Shoulders/ Arms/ Back	Overhead Press, Single-arm front raise, pull-ups and chin-ups, barbell curls, single-arm dumbbell curls, bent-over barbell row, V-grip lat pulldown and single-arm seated cable row (max 8)	15-60 minutes (ex: jump rope)	8000 steps	X	X
SATURDAY	X	X	15-60 minutes (ex: stair climbing)	8000 steps	X	X
SUNDAY	X	X	X	8000 steps	X	10 minutes of full body stretching

ReShapeHER 3-Day Fitness Plan | Week 4						
	RESISTANCE TRAINING AREA OF FOCUS	**RESISTANCE TRAINING LIFTS (15-60 MINUTES)**	**CARDIO**	**NEAT**	**PROGRESSIVE OVERLOAD**	**FLEXIBILITY**
MONDAY	Abs/Glutes	Bulgarian Split Squats, Weighted Step-ups, Hip Abduction/ Adduction, Reverse Glute hyper, Bear Crawl, Single-leg Deadift, Seated Russian twist, Cable Ab pulldown (max 8)	15-60 minutes (ex: Bike ride)	8000 steps	no more than <10% every 4 weeks (70-85% RPM for beginner, 70-100% for advanced)	X
TUESDAY	X	X	X	8000 steps	X	10 minutes of full body stretching
WEDNES-DAY	Thighs/ Hamstrings	Romanian Deadlift, Alternating Weighted step-ups, walking lunges, Leg press, seated/lying leg curls, cable side leg raises, cable pull-throughs, monster band walks (max 8)	15-60 minutes (ex: planned walk)	8000 steps	X	X
THURSDAY	X	X	X (optional)	8000 steps	X	X
FRIDAY	Shoulders/ Arms/ Back	Push-ups, single-arm lateral raise, cable press-downs, kettlebell swings, single-arm tricep push-downs, inverted row, single-arm seated cable row, single-arm lat pulldown and straight-arm cable pulldown (max 8)	15-60 minutes (ex: ellipti-cal machine)	8000 steps	X	X
SATURDAY	X	X	15-60 minutes (ex: pilates)	8000 steps	X	X
SUNDAY	X	X	X	8000 steps	X	10 minutes of full body stretching

ReShapeHER Fitness Plan Key	
Order of Exercise	— Resistance Training Before Cardio — Large Muscle Groups before smaller ones
Sets per Resistance Training lift	3-4 Maximum
Repetitions per Resistance Training lift	8-15 Maximum
Tempo per Resistance Training lift	3:1:2 to 4:2:3 (in seconds)
Intensity per Resistance Training lift	— 70% 1RPM (1 rep maximum) for beginners — 70-85% for intermediate lifters — 70-100% for advanced lifters
Rest time between lifts	—1-2 minutes for lower intensity lifts —2-3 minutes for higher intensity lifts
Rest time between muscle groups	48 hours minimum
Recommended time for Resistance Training and/or Cardio Sessions	—15 minutes minimum —60 minutes maximum
Recommended NEAT	8,000 total daily steps or 56,000 weekly steps
Recommended flexibility goal	20 total minutes per week (full-body)

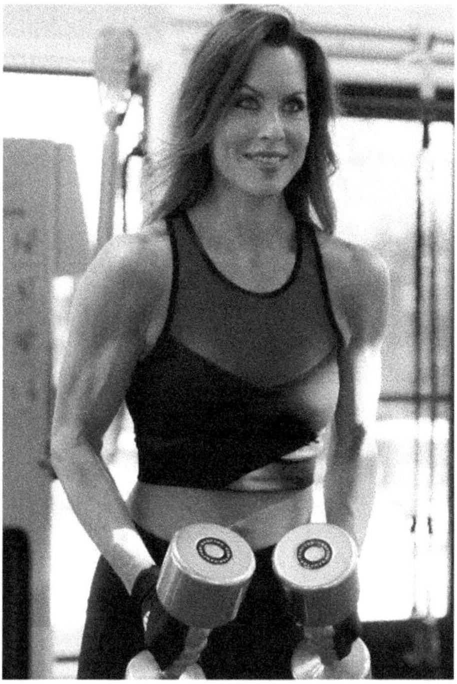

WHEN TO SWITCH FROM 3-DAY TO 5-DAY

If a mother would like to advance further with her fitness, find more time in her schedule, and want to see even greater results, she would then consider the ReShapeHER 5-Day Fitness Plan.

However, prior to switching from the 3-Day Fitness Plan to the 5-Day Fitness Plan, I would recommend that all aspects of the 3-Day Fitness Plan are maximized prior to doing this. The 5-Day Fitness Plan is intended for mothers with more advanced fitness levels, in that it adds an additional resistance training day to further challenge muscle groups. This 5-Day Fitness Plan allows a mother an additional day to exercise a muscle group she'd like to have a greater emphasis on (abs/glutes, thighs/hamstrings or shoulders/arm/back) to reach her body composition goals. This 5-Day Fitness Plan still allows for a rest day (with NEAT only movements recommended). However, because of the additional day it incorporates for resistance training, it allows for a lesser amount of time for each muscle group to rest.

ReShapeHER 5-Day Fitness Plan

Time Commitment Per Week

Minimum: Five 15 min. sessions of resistance training per week, five 15 min sessions of Cardio per week (can be traded for NEAT when needed), seven days of 8,000 steps of movement per week (totaling 56,000 steps that can be spread throughout the week), and 20 min of full body stretching per week.

Average: Five 30 min. sessions of resistance training per week, five 30 min sessions of cardio per week (can be traded for NEAT when needed), seven days of 8,000 steps of movement per week (totaling 56,000 steps that can be spread throughout the week), and 20 min of full body stretching per week.

Advanced: Five-six 60 min. sessions of resistance training per week (taking advantage of "optional" session), five-six 60 min. sessions of cardio (can be traded for NEAT when needed), seven days of 8,000 steps of movement per week (totaling 56,000 steps that can be spread throughout the week), and 20 min of full body stretching per week.

EAT (Planned Exercise—Resistance Training and Cardio)

For resistance training, the ReShapeHER 5-Day Fitness Plan allows for muscle group(s) to be exercised more than once per week (Abs/Glutes and Thighs/Hamstrings are programmed twice, however these muscle groups can be interchanged for the other two). For each planned workout, 50% time contribution will be spent towards resistance training for days that it is programmed. (For example, for a 1 hour workout, at least 30 minutes would be paid to resistance training). Resistance training should include a 50/50 split of compound and isolation exercises for muscle group(s) listed equaling eight total lifts per muscle group(s) for that day, (with compound lifts being the priority as they require more muscle engagement and should be done first and also prioritized over Isolation ones). For example, on Day 1 for abs/glutes, that would total a maximum of four total lifts for abdominals (2 compound and 2 isolation) and four lifts for glutes (2 compound and 2 isolation). *Day 4 (Shoulders/Arms/Back) is the only day is the only day that has three muscle groups, which would make the compound lift total less than two per muscle group, as three muscle groups are being considered versus two.* Not every planned session will include all the lifts in either the compound or isolation categories, therefore, the lifts can be rotated throughout sessions. In the case of the 5-Day Fitness Plan, all of the lifts for each muscle group can be successfully rotated within the week except the shoulders/arms/back which aren't repeated within the week. This will result in all lifts for this particular muscle group being accomplished within a two week period of time. Lastly, the ReShapeHER 5-Day Fitness Plan recommends a minimum of 15 minutes of resistance training to a maximum of 60 minutes per planned session.

Resistance Training Equipment Needed

Gym Membership or Home Equipment listed below:

ReShapeHER Program Home Equipment Needs
Dumbbells
Medicine Ball or Heavy Duffle Bag
Resistance Bands - looped and open
Sturdy Chair/Table
Hanging Bar (or playground equipment)
Floor mat

Progressive Overload is included with the ReShapeHER program, as it recommends practicing it no more than <10% every 2-4 weeks (70-85% RPM for beginner, 70-100% for advanced). A mother can choose to maximize this practice, should she want to grow her lean muscle tissue to a greater degree depending on her season.

Planned cardiovascular exercises are programmed 6x/week in this plan (with one optional day), and one rest day built in. These exercises will be done second to resistance training for days where both are scheduled. Cardiovascular exercises should include the ones that a mother enjoys and one type isn't preferred over another. LISS (low-intensity, steady state) cardio or HIIT can be performed with this plan, depending on what a mother prefers (as both will support her fitness goals). The ReShapeHER program recommends a minimum of 15 minutes of cardiovascular exercises to a maximum of 60 minutes per planned session.

NEAT (unplanned exercise)

The ReShapeHER program recommends a step tracker for these unplanned movements a mother can achieve just by having an active lifestyle. They should be counted separately from their EAT, however, on days that a mother may not have time to complete her EAT, she can replace them with her NEAT activities (knowing this will decrease her caloric output potential). This program also includes a minimum daily step count of 8,000 steps (even on rest days).

Cardio requirements

Step counter/tracker for NEAT and EAT

Stretching Requirements

Floor mats

Nutrition

The ReShapeHER program recommends a mother use the calculator to determine her TDEE (based on her individual values), to understand the amount of calories and macronutrients she needs to consume, depending on her season. This TDEE should be recalculated, and possibly adjusted every 2-4 weeks based on a mother's weight and activity levels.

RESHAPEHER 5-DAY OUTLINE

Fitness Portion:

Day 1	Abs/Glutes + LISS or HIIT cardio + NEAT
Day 2	Thighs/Hamstrings + LISS or HIIT cardio + NEAT
Day 3	LISS or HIIT cardio (optional) + NEAT + Flexibility
Day 4	Shoulders/Arms/Back + LISS or HIIT cardio + NEAT
Day 5	Abs/Glutes (can be interchanged) + LISS or HIIT cardio + NEAT
Day 6	Thighs/Hamstrings (can be interchanged) + LISS or HIIT cardio + NEAT
Day 7	REST + NEAT + Flexibility

RESISTANCE TRAINING (EAT): 15 minutes minimum on recommended days; maximum 60 minutes (50% time contribution of total workout). Lifts are split 50/50 by choosing half compound and half isolation for each given muscle group (8 lifts maximum).

Progressive overload: no more than <10% every 4 weeks (70-85% RPM for beginner, 70-100% for advanced)

CARDIO (EAT): 15 minutes minimum on recommended days; should follow resistance training when combined with it; maximum 60 min.

LISS or HIIT (low-intensity or high-intensity) Can be replaced with NEAT

NEAT: Accomplished as an addition to EAT in order to reach daily minimum step goal of 8,000

FLEXIBILITY: 20 minutes full-body stretching requirements per week

REST DAY: No planned Resistance Training or Cardio; includes NEAT goal of 8000 steps

NUTRITION: TDEE based on season and followed; recalculated and possibly adjusted every 2-4 weeks depending on weight and/or activity levels

ReShapeHER 5-Day Fitness Plan | Week 1

	RESISTANCE TRAINING AREA OF FOCUS	RESISTANCE TRAINING LIFTS (15-60 MINUTES)	CARDIO	NEAT	PROGRESSIVE OVERLOAD	FLEXIBILITY
MONDAY	Abs/Glutes	Back Squats, Sumo Deadlift, Hip Thrusts, Cable kick-back, Suitcase Deadlift, Medicine Ball slams, Abdominal Crunches, Hanging Knee Raise/ Twist, (max 8)	15-60 minutes (ex: run)	8000 steps	no more than <10% every 4 weeks (70-85% RPM for beginner, 70-100% for advanced)	X
TUESDAY	Thighs/ Hamstrings	Romanian Deadlift, Alternating Weighted step-ups, walking lunges, Leg press, seated/lying leg curls, cable side leg raises, cable pull-throughs, monster band walks (max 8)	15-60 minutes (HIIT circuit using body weight such as jumping jacks, burpees, etc)	8000 steps	X	X
WEDNES-DAY	X	X	X (optional)	8000 steps	X	10 minutes of full body stretching
THURSDAY	Shoulders/ Arms/ Back	Overhead Press, Single-arm front raise, pull-ups and chin-ups, barbell curls, single-arm dumbbell curls, bent-over barbell row, V-grip lat pulldown and single-arm seated cable row (max 8)	15-60 minutes (ex: planned brisk walk or hike)	8000 steps	X	X
FRIDAY	Abs/Glutes	Bulgarian Split Squats, Weighted step-ups, Hip Abduction/ Adduction, Reverse Glute hyper, Bear Crawl, Single-leg Deadlift, Seated Russian twist, Cable Ab pulldown (max 8)	15-60 minutes (ex: row)	8000 steps	X	X
SATURDAY	Thighs/ Hamstrings	Romanian Deadlift, Alternating Weighted step-ups, walking lunges, Leg press, seated/lying leg curls, cable side leg raises, cable pull-throughs, monster band walks (max 8)	15-60 minutes (ex: spin class or bike ride)	8000 steps	X	X
SUNDAY	X	X	X	8000 steps	X	10 minutes of full body stretching

ReShapeHER 5-Day Fitness Plan | Week 2

	RESISTANCE TRAINING AREA OF FOCUS	RESISTANCE TRAINING LIFTS (15-60 MINUTES)	CARDIO	NEAT	PROGRESSIVE OVERLOAD	FLEXIBILITY
MONDAY	Abs/Glutes	Back Squats, Sumo Deadlift, Hip Thrusts, Cable kick-back, Suitcase Deadlift, Medicine Ball slams, Abdominal Crunches, Hanging Knee Raise/ Twist, (max 8)	15-60 minutes (ex: hike)	8000 steps	no more than <10% every 4 weeks (70-85% RPM for beginner, 70-100% for advanced)	X
TUESDAY	Thighs/ Hamstrings	Romanian Deadlift, Alternating Weighted step-ups, walking lunges, Leg press, seated/lying leg curls, cable side leg raises, cable pull-throughs, monster band walks (max 8)	15-60 minutes (ex: HIIT circuit using body weight - such as jumping jacks, burpees, etc.)	8000 steps	X	X
WEDNES-DAY	X	X	X (optional)	8000 steps	X	10 minutes of full body stretching
THURSDAY	Shoulders/ Arms/ Back	Push-ups, Single-arm lateral raise, Cable press-downs, Kettlebell swings, Single-arm tricep push-downs, Inverted row, Single-arm seated cable row, Single-arm lateral pulldown and Straight-arm cable pulldown	15-60 minutes (ex: planned brisk walk or hike)	8000 steps	X	X
FRIDAY	Abs/Glutes	Bulgarian Split Squats, Weighted step-ups, Hip Abduction/ Adduction, Reverse Glute hyper, Bear Crawl, Single-leg Deadlift, Seated Russian twist, Cable Ab pulldown (max 8)	15-60 minutes (ex: brisk walk)	8000 steps	X	X
SATURDAY	Thighs/ Hamstrings	Romanian Deadlift, Alternating Weighted step-ups, walking lunges, Leg press, seated/lying leg curls, cable side leg raises, cable pull-throughs, monster band walks (max 8)	15-60 minutes (ex: swim)	8000 steps	X	X
SUNDAY	X	X	X	8000 steps	X	10 minutes of full body stretching

ReShapeHER 5-Day Fitness Plan | Week 3

	RESISTANCE TRAINING AREA OF FOCUS	RESISTANCE TRAINING LIFTS (15-60 MINUTES)	CARDIO	NEAT	PROGRESSIVE OVERLOAD	FLEXIBILITY
MONDAY	Abs/Glutes	Back Squats, Sumo Deadlift, Hip Thrusts, Cable kick-back, Suitcase Deadlift, Medicine Ball slams, Abdominal Crunches, Hanging Knee Raise/ Twist, (max 8)	15-60 minutes (ex: run)	8000 steps	no more than <10% every 4 weeks (70-85% RPM for beginner, 70-100% for advanced)	X
TUESDAY	Thighs/ Hamstrings	Romanian Deadlift, Alternating Weighted step-ups, walking lunges, Leg press, seated/lying leg curls, cable side leg raises, cable pull-throughs, monster band walks (max 8)	15-60 minutes (ex: HIIT circuit using body weight - such as jumping jacks, burpees, etc.)	8000 steps	X	X
WEDNESDAY	X	X	X (optional)	8000 steps	X	10 minutes of full body stretching
THURSDAY	Shoulders/ Arms/ Back	Overhead Press, Single-arm front raise, Pull-ups and Chin-ups, Barbell curls, Single-arm Dumbbell curls, Bent-over barbell row, V-grip lat pulldown and Single-arm seated Cable Row (max 8)	15-60 minutes (ex: planned brisk walk or hike)	8000 steps	X	X
FRIDAY	Abs/Glutes	Bulgarian Split Squats, Weighted step-ups, Hip Abduction/ Adduction, Reverse Glute hyper, Bear Crawl, Single-leg Deadlift, Seated Russian twist, Cable Ab pulldown (max 8)	15-60 minutes (ex: row)	8000 steps	X	X
SATURDAY	Thighs/ Hamstrings	Romanian Deadlift, Alternating Weighted step-ups, walking lunges, Leg press, seated/lying leg curls, cable side leg raises, cable pull-throughs, monster band walks (max 8)	15-60 minutes (ex: spin class or bike ride)	8000 steps	X	X
SUNDAY	X	X	X	8000 steps	X	10 minutes of full body stretching

ReShapeHER 5-Day Fitness Plan | Week 4						
	RESISTANCE TRAINING AREA OF FOCUS	**RESISTANCE TRAINING LIFTS (15-60 MINUTES)**	**CARDIO**	**NEAT**	**PROGRESSIVE OVERLOAD**	**FLEXIBILITY**
MONDAY	Abs/Glutes	Back Squats, Sumo Deadlift, Hip Thrusts, Cable kick-back, Suitcase Deadlift, Medicine Ball slams, Abdominal Crunches, Hanging Knee Raise/ Twist, (max 8)	15-60 minutes (ex: hike)	8000 steps	no more than <10% every 4 weeks (70-85% RPM for beginner, 70-100% for advanced)	X
TUESDAY	Thighs/ Hamstrings	Romanian Deadlift, Alternating Weighted step-ups, walking lunges, Leg press, seated/lying leg curls, cable side leg raises, cable pull-throughs, monster band walks (max 8)	15-60 minutes (ex: HIIT circuit using body weight - such as jumping jacks, burpees, etc.)	8000 steps	X	X
WEDNES-DAY	X	X	X (optional)	8000 steps	X	10 minutes of full body stretching
THURSDAY	Shoulders/ Arms/ Back	Push-ups, Single-arm lateral raise, Cable press-downs, Kettlebell swings, Single-arm tricep push-downs, Inverted row, Single-arm seated Cable row, Single-arm lat pulldowns and Straight-arm cable pulldown (max 8)	15-60 minutes (ex: planned brisk walk or hike)	8000 steps	X	X
FRIDAY	Abs/Glutes	Bulgarian Split Squats, Weighted step-ups, Hip Abduction/ Adduction, Reverse Glute hyper, Bear Crawl, Single-leg Deadlift, Seated Russian twist, Cable Ab pulldown (max 8)	15-60 minutes (ex: brisk walk)	8000 steps	X	X
SATURDAY	Thighs/ Hamstrings	Romanian Deadlift, Alternating Weighted step-ups, walking lunges, Leg press, seated/lying leg curls, cable side leg raises, cable pull-throughs, monster band walks (max 8)	15-60 minutes (ex: swim)	8000 steps	X	X
SUNDAY	X	X	X	8000 steps	X	10 minutes of full body stretching

ReShapeHER Fitness Plan Key	
Order of Exercise	— Resistance Training Before Cardio — Large Muscle Groups before smaller ones
Sets per Resistance Training lift	3-4 Maximum
Repetitions per Resistance Training lift	8-15 Maximum
Tempo per Resistance Training lift	3:1:2 to 4:2:3 (in seconds)
Intensity per Resistance Training lift	— 70% 1RPM (1 rep maximum) for beginners — 70-85% for intermediate lifters — 70-100% for advanced lifters
Rest time between lifts	—1-2 minutes for lower intensity lifts —2-3 minutes for higher intensity lifts
Rest time between muscle groups	48 hours minimum
Recommended time for Resistance Training and/ or Cardio Sessions	—15 minutes minimum —60 minutes maximum
Recommended NEAT	8,000 total daily steps or 56,000 weekly steps
Recommended flexibility goal	20 total minutes per week (full-body)

PUTTING IT ALL TOGETHER – THE RESHAPEHER 3-DAY AND 5-DAY FITNESS PLANS

The ReShapeHER program recommends all mothers that are beginners or have taken time away from their fitness, start with the 3-Day Fitness Plan and advance to the 5-Day Fitness Plan only when they feel that they have developed the muscle and cardiovascular strength to do so. This advancement should only be made once they have maximized all aspects of the 3-Day Fitness Plan, including some time spent applying Progressive Overload to their lifts. The 3-Day Fitness Plan allows for each muscle group to be exercised once per week, 5 days of programmed cardio (with one day being optional) and a NEAT step count of 8,000. NEAT is not optional on any day of the week in order to promote an active and healthy lifestyle.

The 5-Day Fitness Plan is built more for the mother who is more advanced in fitness, as it has a recommended five days of resistance training, allowing for two muscle groups to be repeated each week. *It is recommended to repeat Abs/Glutes for Day 5 and Thighs/Hamstrings for Day 6, however, these can be changed to another muscle group. However, it is critical that when selecting it is critical that when selecting a muscle group of choice for days 5 and 6, a mother exercises a muscle group that has rested for a minimum of 48 hours.* There are six cardio days recommended in the 5-Day Fitness Plan (with one being optional) and a NEAT step count of 8,000. NEAT is also not an option any day of the week in order to promote an active and healthy lifestyle.

How to Split Up Planned Exercises

Should a mother choose to split up the resistance training and cardio activities on any particular day, this can be done as long as she prioritizes the resistance training portion. This is because, as mothers with busy schedules, should the day get away from us and we don't have time to complete the second portion of our fitness plan for the day, the resistance piece has been done (which is the greatest contributor to muscle strength/growth and body composition overall). Also, if the resistance portion is done first, it enables us to use our greatest amount of energy and focus (which is most likely during the first half of the day versus the second) to successfully accomplish lifts with the greatest form and execution. Resistance and cardio can also be split up by doing the resistance portion only (in case there isn't time allotted for the cardio piece on a particular day), and the cardio piece can be made up on the "optional" day if need be. It is critical that if a mother wants to experience the full benefits that the ReShapeHER program can deliver, that she fulfills the recommended resistance training and cardio portions that are established in the plan.

Should a planned cardio session be missed in the ReShapeHER

program, this can be substituted by staying active and focusing on our NEAT, as this program understands that the contribution of our weekly NEAT is 15% of our overall daily caloric contribution! Although it isn't recommended to make a habit out of missing our cardiovascular activities, life happens and the ReShapeHER program allows any mother to be able to adapt. This program not only puts an emphasis on the importance of a mother living an active and healthy lifestyle in order to achieve her goals, but also motivates her to do so, helping her understand the importance of her daily NEAT levels.

Switching from the 3-Day to 5-Day Fitness Plan and Vise-Versa

Regardless of the plan a mother chooses with ReShapeHER, it can be tailored to her individual needs. For example, if she's a beginner, she can choose to exercise the 3-Day Fitness Plan, moving to the 5-Day Fitness Plan when she feels like she's built up her fitness level. If she is a busy mother with limited time to dedicate to fitness, she can start with the 3-Day Fitness Plan, and maximize it, before moving to the 5-Day Fitness Plan at a later time when her schedule or fitness level permits. Let's say she's a mother who has been practicing the 5-Day Fitness Plan and suddenly finds herself in a busy situation; she can always revert back to the 3-Day Fitness Plan to support her fitness progress and then switch back to the 5-Day Fitness Plan at a later point.

Tailoring Your Plan Based on Your Time Availability

In addition to a mother being able to maximize the ReShapeHER 3-Day or 5-Day Fitness Plans based on her time commitments, she can also maximize each plan based on the fitness efforts she is able to contribute throughout the week. For example, should she only have time for the 3-Day Fitness Plan, on the days during the week that she can maximize her time, she can choose to do exercises that require more of this time and possibly more exertion. For example, she may choose to do additional compound lifts or apply more towards her Progressive Overload practices (not to exceed the recommended 60 minutes per day). She may also choose to tack on more time for her cardiovascular activities (not to exceed the recommended 60 minutes) and NEAT (tracking more steps) in order to contribute more toward your calorie output and overall fitness health.

When it comes to time in general, the ReShapeHER program understands that time can often be limited, especially with busy mothers! This understanding is built into both the 3-Day and 5-Day Fitness Plans. With limited time, a busy mother can switch from the 5-Day Fitness Plan to the 3-Day Fitness Plan as mentioned above, trade a suggested day for another, increase NEAT levels if EAT is lessened, switch LISS cardio for HIIT movements if doing the 5-Day Fitness Plan with an advanced fitness level, maximize her efforts with Progressive Overload to make more progress within the time constraints she has, etc. Also, with limited time, a mother can prioritize compound lifts in lieu of isolation ones that will offer more muscle recruitment or repeat them with specific muscle groups. By practicing the ReShapeHER program consistently over time a mother does have, she will be able to understand which lifts are making the greatest contributions to her ideal body composition.

Maintaining Muscle Growth

The beauty of the ReShapeHER program is that a busy mother can successfully switch from the 5-Day Fitness Plan to the 3-Day one, and still maintain her lean muscle tissue over a few months. This idea is supported by scientific evidence of strength training volume, mainly frequency, that was conducted in the 1988 Graves et al study, "Effect of reduced training frequency on muscular strength." In his study, he concluded that "strength values for subjects who reduced training to 2 and 1 days per week were not significantly different ($p \geq 0.05$) from post-training strength values." The data suggested that "muscular strength can be maintained for up to 12 weeks with reduced training frequency."[45] Therefore, should a mother experience a time in which she's busy and cannot exercise the 5-Day Fitness Plan, she can do the 3-Day Fitness Plan knowing that she can at least maintain the muscle growth that she's made with the 5-Day Fitness Plan for a few months, allowing her the flexibility to balance her lifestyle and then switch back at a future date. When a mother then decides to switch back to the 5-Day Fitness Plan, she can then make contributions to her muscle growth once again, as her resistance training efforts will become more frequent and she can also apply the practices of Progressive Overload.

Tailoring Your Plan to Your Season

Tailoring the ReShapeHER program goes even further than just with time, in that you can also tailor it to the season you may be in. If you've decided you need to be in an "off" season for a while and are practicing the 3-Day Fitness Plan, you can switch to the 5-Day Fitness Plan to allow for your muscle groups to be more challenged throughout the week. Maybe you've decided to enter an "on" season in which you switch from the 5-Day Fitness Plan to the 3-Day Fitness Plan as your goal becomes less about muscle growth and more about fat loss, as you make efforts toward your overall calorie output. You may decide to do this 3-Day Fitness Plan (with an increase in both cardio and NEAT) to allow for this additional calorie output, with the continued three days of resistance training that continues to support the muscle growth you've made in your prior "off" season. The options are endless with the ReShapeHER program when it comes to being any type of mother and wanting to achieve a great body composition!

How To Make Up For A Missed Day

Should a busy mom miss a day with the ReShapeHER program, she can simply trade it for another day (keeping in mind that it is recommended to have a 48-hour break between training any specific muscle group). Therefore, if she trades the missed day for another day and her schedule reflects back-to-back days of resistance training, she will need to make sure she is training two different types of muscle groups. She will also keep in mind that many compound movements train muscle groups collectively, so it will behoove her to also make sure she isn't doing the same compound movements for these back-to-back days.

HOW TO MEASURE YOUR FITNESS RESULTS WITH THE RESHAPEHER PROGRAM

Making improvements to one's body composition is a process that takes time and consistency that can't be measured accurately from just reading a scale that gives us a body weight value only. Remember, you can't change your body composition to obtain an ideal "toned" state with your body as a mother, unless you make improvements to not only your body fat but also your lean muscle tissue. As I've discussed in previous chapters, as mothers we have often made the mistake of contributing efforts to lose body fat alone, but not making these same efforts to maintain or grow our muscle. For these reasons, our body composition goals have not been met.

I've discussed in previous chapters, how muscle development is a process that takes time and is affected by factors such as body size, composition, hormones, muscle response, resistance put on the muscle, how frequently this is done, the amount of time for recovery, the amounts and types of macronutrients the body is given, etc. These are a lot of factors to consider, however, the ReShapeHER program has thought this all out for you! With either the 3-Day or 5-Day Fitness Plans, a mother can put her best efforts forward to effectively develop her muscle and lose body fat, allowing her to have positive, measurable results in a short period of time.

Although there can be no exact prediction on how long it will take for a mother to reach her ultimate body composition goal, she can start seeing long-term results in as little as 4-6 weeks with the ReShapeHER program regardless of her starting point. *(Mothers who have practiced this program have demonstrated these results!)*

The longer a mother consistently practices the ReShapeHER program, the more dramatic the results she will experience over time in doing so. In lieu of just using a scale to determine her fitness results, a mother that has been educated with the ReShapeHER program information, will learn how to effectively interpret her results with body composition data. This data will give her insight on the two factors (body fat and muscle mass) that are the most important, when not only determining her body composition but her overall state of health.

There are many options of scales on the market that can give a mother accessibility to this type of data. One of which includes a Bioelectrical Impedance Analysis (BIA). This BIA sends very low, safe electrical signals through the feet and into the body. This signal meets resistance when it hits fat tissue and passes quickly through water in the body. This resistance is what the device uses to determine body composition measurements. There are other tools available in the marketplace that measure body composition data that are slightly more accurate (DEXA, hydrostatic, etc); however, they are usually much more expensive. Usually, most gyms and fitness centers offer the ability for a mother to quickly do a body comp test if she has a membership or is willing to pay a nominal fee for a test. There are also many other types that can be used at home and linked to your phone. This type of BIA scale is highly encouraged with the ReShapeHER program so a mother is able to track her body fat and lean muscle tissue in lieu of just her overall body weight!

Being familiar with this data as a mother progresses through her fitness journey, provides her much greater insight into her efforts and overall composition versus just using a body weight scale. I've discussed this in previous chapters, but when a mother focuses on growing and maintaining her muscle, she can prevent falls and illnesses and possibly improve her metabolism. This is especially important to understand because as mothers, we lose this muscle over time with poor diets, the aging process, and many other reasons discussed in this book. Additionally, if our fat mass is too great, this can also lead us to many illnesses such as hypertension, strokes, and cardiovascular disease.

Values that contribute to our overall body composition, such as water and bone mass, are also important for mothers to take note of. As mothers, if we practice a fitness plan with a diet rich in whole foods and movements that include resistance training, we can maintain our bone mass, helping us reduce the risk of osteoporosis. Our total percentage of water that's found inside (intracellular) and outside (extracellular) of our cells can give us insight into our state of hydration. Our extracellular water, should it be high, may be indicative of heart, liver, malnutrition, or kidney disease.

According to the article *Body Cardio – What are the normal ranges for body composition?* [46] the following chart can be used as a benchmark to determine normal ranges for body composition data. Keep in mind that body composition scales provide information for many data points, but the ones mentioned below are the primary ones you will need to understand as they make up your total body composition.

WOMEN'S BODY COMPOSITION		
Water Mass	All ages	45-60%
Bone Mass	All ages	2.5-4%
Fat Mass (Body fat %, not BMI)	Ages 20–39	22-33%
	Ages 40–59	24-34%
	Ages 60–79	25-36%
Muscle Mass	Ages 20-39	63-75.5%
	Ages 40-59	62-73.5%
	Ages 60-79	60-72.5%

Once a mother familiarizes herself with her body composition data, she can then familiarize herself with the process of tracking her efforts as they relate to this data over the course of her fitness journey. She will be able to understand how changes in both her fitness movements and nutrition play a part in supporting her unique body composition. She will have a better idea of understanding where she needs to make changes. All of these insights give her greater control over her fitness efforts that a home scale simply cannot provide and gives her ultimate **CONTROL** in understanding her fitness efforts with the ReShapeHER program!

It is critical for all mothers to remember that our bodies don't operate in a vacuum as they are always in a constant state of flux. Numbers and values are only part of our health picture and change over time. The key to overall good health is making sure that we are consistently practicing good habits that benefit all aspects of our being, as we continue in our fitness journey. Through the consistent practice of the ReShapeHER program and a mindfulness of our overall health, we can all reach her fitness goals over a short time!

ALWAYS REMEMBER YOUR WHY!

As you begin or continue your fitness journey, always remember the "glue" that will keep you moving in the directions of your goals—your WHY! There will be many days that you won't feel motivated. . .remember motivation is fleeting. We, as mothers, cannot rely on it to carry us through our journey. Our consistency and dedication to the soul-driven reason why we started our journey, are the things that will bring us success. Hold on to your WHY, cherish it and revisit it often. Always continue to ask yourself what would happen if you didn't fulfill your WHY. This answer will most often be the only reason you need to lace up your shoes and make it happen!

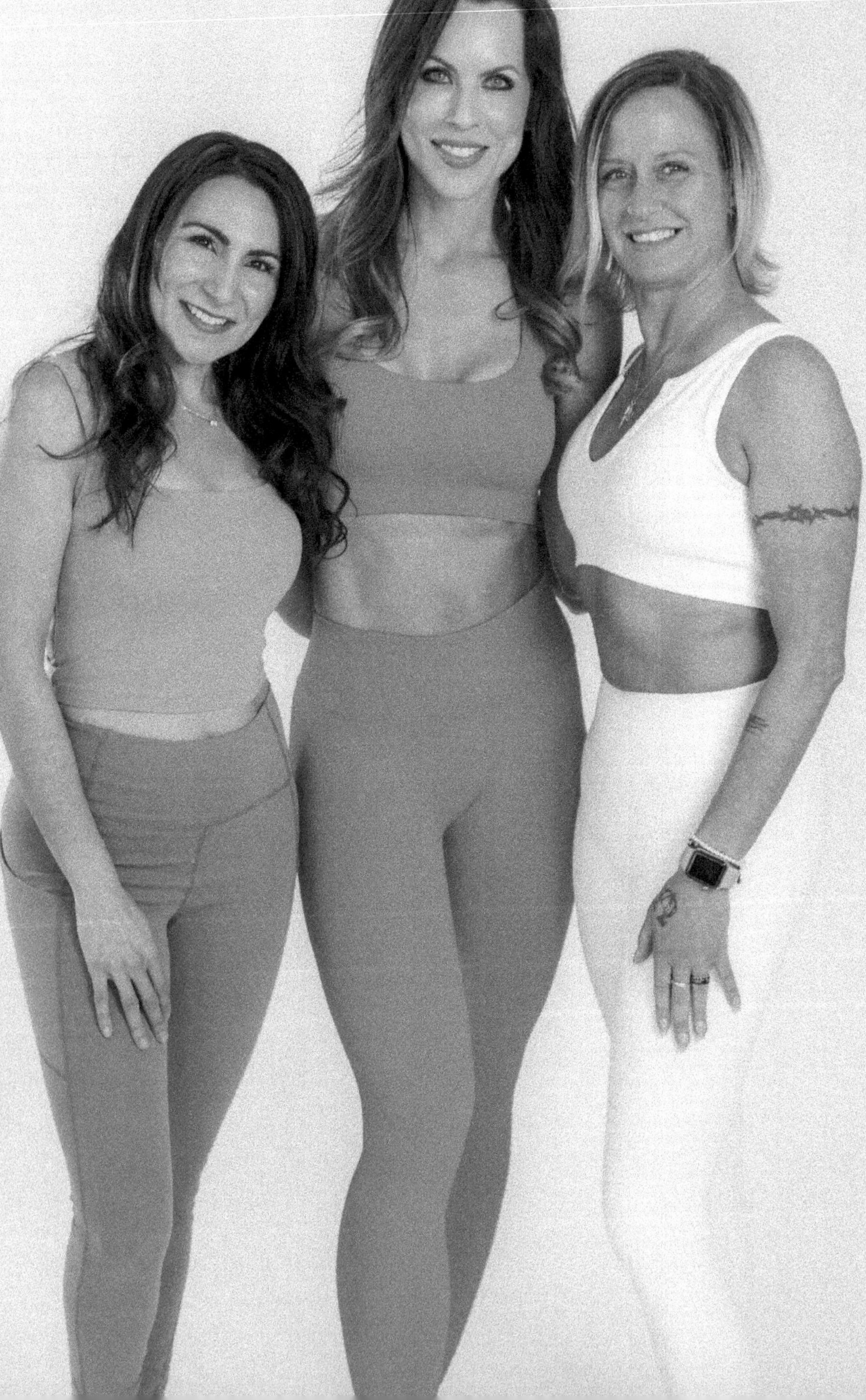

13

Maintaining Your ReShapeHER Physique

(aka: "Maintenance" season)

ONCE YOU ACHIEVE YOUR DESIRED body composition with the ReShapeHER program, maintaining it is just as important! By this point, you'll understand that through the consistent practices this program has to offer, you'll ultimately have the control to ensure that your body remains healthy and fit through the ebbs and flows of life and challenges that will present themselves along the way. You will know that maintaining a fit physique requires the knowledge of how to "trust the process" and be confident in the steps you'll need to take in order to achieve your individualized balance. You will learn to appreciate how you will be able to continue to tailor the ReShapeHER program to your fitness goals as you evolve. With this program, your body will continue to achieve greater levels of fitness even during your "maintenance" seasons, allowing you to enjoy your fitness journey and reach plateaus you never thought you could before.

As I've discussed in previous chapters, your "maintenance" seasons will serve one of two purposes:

1. To serve as a temporary period of time in which you take a "diet

break" from a calorie deficit ("on" season) or a break from a calorie surplus ("off" season)

2. To serve as your "status quo" period, in which you simply practice your fitness plan with consistency, not having a goal of either gaining or losing body fat and supporting your body composition with a good diet that suffices your TDEE

A long and healthy maintenance season should actually be the goal for mothers. Being able to achieve a maintenance season with a healthy body composition that you enjoy, can be one of your greatest accomplishments. It can boost your confidence and allow you to share this confidence with other fellow mothers. How successfully you practice the healthy habits you've learned with the ReShapeHER program, allows you to decide how long you can remain in this period. Regardless of what circumstances life might throw at you as a mother, the ReShapeHER program will provide you the ability to work your way back to a successful "maintenance" season.

MAINTAINING YOUR RESHAPEHER BODY WITH LITTLE TIME

Thinking of a fitness plan in terms of smaller steps can be extremely effective when incorporating it into your life and working toward your long-term goals. Oftentimes as mothers, when we think of all of the steps we would need to take to reach a goal, it can seem overwhelming and may discourage us from even pursuing it because of the amount of time we know has to be dedicated to doing it. Metabolizing goals on a smaller scale can be very effective in terms of driving motivation and our ability to start practicing habits that collectively will lead us to our long-term goals. Goals, whether big or small, can be easily managed with the ReShapeHER program. This program allows any mother to tailor it to her lifestyle, in order to reach her goals. Additionally, it gives a mother insights into how she can speed up her progress if her time becomes more available. The great thing about the ReShapeHER program, is that regardless of a mother's time dedication, she can successfully reach her body composition goals as long as she practices it consistently.

Flexibility with the ReShapeHER Program

With the ReShapeHER program, a mother can make a decision based on her time commitments, by practicing either the 3-Day or 5-Day Fitness Plans. She could even switch back and forth, depending on her time commitment each week/month. She could split up her EAT (planned exercises), put them on different days, or even trade them for NEAT (unplanned exercises). She could make better use of her time doing her EAT, by maximizing her applications of Progressive Overload with her resistance training. She could make greater efforts towards her body composition with fat loss, by utilizing the ReShapeHER calculator and setting her goals with her macronutrients, making an even greater contribution with her diet, should she not have as much time for her planned exercise. She could also make greater contributions with her overall movement, by taking advantage of her NEAT. With the ReShapeHER program, a mother ultimately has an outline to allow her to put her best foot forward when it comes to little time, yet still being able to achieve her fitness goals.

My "Onion" Analogy

Personally, the way I think of a goal is like the layers of an onion, with my long-term goal being the center. The first layer is my daily goals. These layers get peeled first and start the process of getting to the center in due time. I prioritize my daily goals when it comes to my fitness, making sure I'm checking them off on a daily basis. By making these daily goals, I'm able to zoom in on my daily activities (the following layers of the onion), which collectively allow me to create the habits that lead to my long-term goal. Through daily goals, you are able to make positive adjustments along the way that contribute to successful outcomes. They fulfill the box of instant gratification, in that they help drive satisfaction when they're accomplished. By having smaller, daily goals, we can create palpable commitments to ourselves. Even if they aren't met every day, they allow us room to establish solutions that negate us feeling guilty or doubtful. As we continue to peel the onion in terms of our goals, we work towards the center and eventually reach it with hard work and consistency.

It is critical to remember that with our consistency that's manifested in our daily goals, we are able to make an even greater impact toward our long-term goals. Our weekly goals allow us to build on the habits that bring us to success. Through weekly goals, we are able to negate patterns that derail us, as we gain a greater understanding of patterns that bring us results we desire.

Monthly goals are critical when looking back and getting a better "bird's-eye" view of our progress. They can help us understand more about the progress we are truly making as we can start to see some form of patterns that are being created, and also the time invested in creating them. They also allow us to look forward and make very conservative predictions on how we may fare in terms of a month or two from that point, should the consistency of daily goals be met. After a month of consistently practicing good habits with a solid fitness plan like the ReShapeHER program, we can have an even greater insight into how our efforts have translated into results. We may start to see more visual, aesthetic changes that can fuel our motivation to practice our fitness plans. Through consistent practice, we can determine what impact our nutrition is making and what adjustments need to be made toward our TDEE over time. We can understand what impact our resistance training and cardio are making toward our body composition and when it may be appropriate to further drive these efforts.

Yearly goals give us the greatest viewpoint on our efforts, as they incorporate the daily, weekly, and monthly goals we've made. By analyzing these yearly goals, we can appreciate the progress we've made and the lifelong habits we've developed. As a result, we may be able to analyze the positive changes we've made to our health and fitness, driving our confidence even further. We can start being examples and teachers to others, helping them understand how to live a fit and healthier life through our experiences.

Mothers Need to Prioritize Themselves

When it comes to having little time, and also being a mother, one of the hardest things to do is prioritize ourselves. There's always something to be done and someone to think about. We put ourselves last on the list when it comes to many things, often our own health. Although I think we'd all agree that our health and fitness are very important, we often struggle with the "mommy" guilt that comes along with making the commitments to ourselves. However, we need to remember that prioritizing our own health and fitness is NOT SELFISH. If we aren't filling our buckets with self-love, we can't be good mothers, wives, partners, friends, etc. We can't give our children everything we can, because we simply don't have much to give. We need to find room and learn to prioritize ourselves in this area, knowing that if we don't, we aren't doing ourselves or our families any favors. Without doing this, we'll teach our children to make the same choices, leading them down a path of less optimal health and fitness.

Change is HARD

No one said change is an easy process. Change often requires us to temporarily be in a vulnerable place. It asks us to think of things differently or possibly develop a skill we don't feel comfortable doing. It can force us to face things we've been trying to avoid in our lives. Sometimes it can even hurt our ego, as we have to embrace the fact that during a process of change, we may not feel as courageous. This is all normal and OK. The important thing is that we, as mothers, love ourselves enough to be open to the necessary changes that need to be made in order for us to reach our goals. Without changing what doesn't or hasn't worked, we will never reach our goals. It is easy to blame our lack of wanting to change on the fact that we don't have time. When a change is warranted, time should be prioritized. More often than not, we have been doing something that costs us time, in order to prevent us from making the change. Identify this time deterrent and take advantage of the time it's costing you to make the valuable change you need to in order to reach your goals.

No Excuses

Having good fitness and health requires self-love. Part of exercising this self-love is by being honest with ourselves. Sometimes many of us may struggle to admit that we are often excuse-driven or just outright lazy. When it comes to time, this can be one of the easiest things to think we don't have, especially when we are always busy. However, although we have busy schedules, we do spend a part of our day doing activities that may or may not contribute to our fitness goals. It is important to analyze these, and think about whether they deserve to be prioritized. You may need to ask yourself: Do I have time to watch TV? Do I spend time chatting on the phone with friends? Do I ever get bored during the day? If you've answered yes to at least one of these questions, you have the time to add fitness into your life. Even if an excuse of yours isn't listed above, think about the ones that you're making. Are they credible? Oftentimes, if we just take the time to be honest with ourselves, our answer lies within us. More often than not, we have the ability to carve out some time towards our fitness.

The "Moving Train" Analogy

Regardless of how much or little time you are able to contribute toward your fitness in a given day, any small movement in a positive direction toward your goals is a good thing! It might take you longer to achieve your goals than someone else, but you're still making the daily contributions to move in a forward manner. Just as a moving train, whether going down the tracks at 5 mph or 100 mph, is still rolling forward to the next station, so will your time dedication and consistency bring you toward your goals. You may be like the 5 mph train in terms of how long it takes you to reach your destination, but the important thing is that you remember that with continual movement, you will get there. Here's the thing: If you get discouraged and just outright stop your progression, you will get nowhere. What's better—moving at 5 mph or not at all? I think you get my point. **Every small step and time contribution eventually leads you to your ultimate goal.**

When it comes to time and fitness, it's critical to remember that we are all on our own unique journeys. Some of us have dedicated more time toward it earlier in our lives while others may have started the fitness journey later in their lives. There also may be others who, due to time constraints and/or lack of consistency, aren't as fit as they once were. In life, our time contributions may change and some things may have to take precedence over others. Sometimes you may need to make trade-offs in order to continue practicing good fitness. The important thing is that we are always doing our best to make contributions to our fitness regardless of how much time we have.

When it comes to time, we need to remind ourselves as mothers that practicing good fitness is always time well spent, regardless of how much time we have to do it. Through fitness, we can practice one of the greatest demonstrations of self-love and be examples for others to do the same. We can be the best version of ourselves, contributing the most to our overall health and longevity. If practicing good fitness was an insurance policy on longevity, would you take the time to invest in it? The answer comes down to YOU.

MAINTAINING YOUR RESHAPEHER BODY DURING YOUR CYCLE

Although there is a lot of evidence to support that exercise can be helpful during your period for various reasons, many mothers find it hard to accomplish during this time of the month. This can be very discouraging for many, as a mother's strength may be influenced by her menstruation cycle. Due to this phenomenon, it may behoove a mother to adjust their resistance training and/or cardio to match their cycles each month. In this chapter, I'll quickly explain how I've successfully done this to ensure I could balance both my difficult menstrual cycles and also practice the ReShapeHER program. *(Note: not all mothers may need to make these adjustments, as period symptoms vary from person to person).*

Many women may benefit from having the fitness portion of this plan, as well as my nutritional plan, mimic that of their monthly cycle. Their fitness efforts can be based on their menstrual phases, as I'll describe below. By doing this, they can take advantage of the days they know they can control their diet better or have stronger performances with their resistance training. Some months may be easier than others and may not require this type of manipulation to their ReShapeHER program, but the beauty of the plan is knowing that if a mother needs to slightly change it due to her cycle, she can do this successfully.

Follicular Phase (Day 1-15)

During the Follicular Phase (in my case, Day 0 of menstruation to about Day 14 or 15), a mother's main focus should be spent on building her strength with resistance training. Because this is the phase of her menstrual cycle that she has the least amount of symptoms and generally feels better (outside of the first couple days of menstruation), she can focus on building and getting stronger in her workouts. She may want to adjust her resistance training to be about 70% resistance training versus 50% on these days versus cardio, to make sure she's making the most out of this time to build. More focus on compound lifts that strengthen more than one muscle group can be done as well as Progressive Overload adjustments.

For cardiovascular activity, she may choose to do more higher-intensity exercises as she may have more energy to accomplish them during the follicular phase. If she's feeling energetic, she may also push her cardiovascular training a little more, considering she will be facing days ahead during her luteal phase that she won't feel like doing this. She may also try to accomplish more non-planned activity (NEAT) in order to further contribute to her caloric output each day. It will behoove her to try to not miss a day of training during her follicular phase since she will be feeling stronger and more energetic.

When it comes to nutrition during the follicular phase, a mother may want to be more strict with her diet, knowing that in her luteal phase (especially during the onset of PMS symptoms), this is much more difficult to accomplish. She may want to think of her nutritional goals in terms of a month, in which she tries to conserve calories toward her daily caloric intake (TDEE) earlier in the month so she can be a little more flexible toward the end of the month in her luteal phase. She will want to be more focused on foods that are higher in fiber content to add to her satiety so she can conserve more calories later in the month. For example, she might have some form of protein with a large salad to keep her full and satisfied. She will need to try to conserve calories, not wasting them on foods that are not nutrient-dense. Conserving these calories can be successfully done by planning ahead, and thinking of TDEE in terms of a monthly goal versus a weekly one.

Luteal Phase

During her luteal phase, her efforts may need to reflect that of a "maintenance" season, with her resistance training, taking advantage of the energy on the days that she has it. Prior to workouts, she'll want to do more stretching and warm-ups to avoid tendon and ligament injuries as joints can be weaker during this phase. She'll want to be careful not to push weights beyond what she was able to do in the follicular phase to avoid injury, and if she's struggling at a maintenance weight and feeling fatigued, reduce the intensity. She may take more time for rest and recovery, possibly adding a complete rest day to her fitness plan should she need it.

For cardio, she'll keep it at a low intensity in order to conserve energy and not cause fatigue. She'll pay special attention to her non-planned exercise (NEAT) and utilize it more often should she not have the energy to complete her cardio portion of my planned exercise workouts. In the luteal phase, she'll need to practice more patience in terms of what she'll be able to do and how much. The utilization of my NEAT movements will become critical during this phase, all of which is outlined and incorporated into the ReShapeHER program.

In terms of nutrition during a mother's luteal phase, she'll want to focus on foods that help with satiety and fuel her energy. She'll add in more complex carbohydrates to fuel her workouts. For example, she may have oats with peanut butter and honey prior to a workout to ensure she has energy to complete it successfully. She'll try to steer clear of foods that are high in sodium to ensure that they don't add to any symptoms of bloating. Additionally, she'll try her best to focus on drinking as much fluid as possible to assist with keeping her water retention at bay. During the luteal phase, she'll need to pay close attention to her nutrition more than the other phases of her cycle. This is where the nutritional part of the ReShapeHER program is key when it comes to a mother hitting her fitness goals during this part of her cycle.

Having a more difficult time during menstruation shouldn't have to derail a mother's fitness progress when she has a successful plan in place like the ReShapeHER program. Although having a difficult menstruation may force a mother to possibly make adjustments and take a little longer to reach her goals, the important thing to remember is that with continual practice and discipline with the ReShapeHER program, her goals can still be met.

MAINTAINING YOUR RESHAPEHER BODY ON VACATION

By practicing the ReShapeHER program, you can book your trip and not worry that your hard work with your fitness will be lost. "Maintenance" season is a realistic season to be in while traveling. It is much easier to track your nutritional intake at maintenance versus trying to be in a deficit and not be able to enjoy certain foods on vacation. You may need to adjust your movements, as your unplanned exercise (NEAT) may need to replace your planned exercise (EAT) depending on your accessibility to fitness equipment or a gym, but this can easily be done with the ReShapeHER program.

Successful Planning for Workouts

The most effective way you can ensure that your workout is achieved is by getting it done first thing in the morning before the food, drinks, weather, and daily activities tire you from considering this idea later in the day. Booking a hotel that you know has a gym or space to do your workouts is key. Packing and ensuring you have enough workout clothes for each day will be critical. You'll want to ensure that your environment reflects that of your fitness goals on vacation. Make sure you build in the time on your vacation to accomplish your goals.

The beauty of the ReShapeHER program is that even during vacation, it can be successfully practiced. For the planned exercise portion, both the 3-Day and 5-Day Fitness Plans include the muscle groups that need to be exercised on certain days to ensure you achieve a full body workout. For either plan, you may choose to switch these days around depending on when you're able to accomplish a workout, as long as you allow for a 48-hour rest period between working out the same muscle group.

For example, with the 3-Day Fitness Plan you may choose to do resistance training on your Abs/Glutes on Day 1, followed by Thighs/Hamstrings on Day 2 (skipping a rest/optional NEAT day in between). You may decide to have all three lift days back-to-back, followed by days of NEAT alone. The important thing is that you are prioritizing the resistance portion of your exercise plan and contributing toward your NEAT by staying active, in order to stay within your TDEE and maintain your body composition.

For the 5-Day Fitness Plan, you have more days incorporated for resistance training, so you may choose to do more days back-to-back or drop down to the 3-Day Fitness Plan if you don't have the time to contribute as many days toward your resistance training as you had hoped. The important thing is that you are doing the same as you would with the 3-Day Fitness Plan in prioritizing resistance training and contributing toward your TDEE in order to maintain your body composition during vacation.

If the gym has limited resistance training items, the ReShapeHER program is easy to follow in that it includes at-home variations for all of the recommended lifts for both the 3-Day and 5-Day Fitness Plans. Depending on your fitness level, the resistance bands may not offer you enough resistance to grow; however, they can certainly allow you to maintain your lean muscle tissue while on vacation. You will just need to select a challenging rep range (based on their resistance) in order to accomplish this.

When it comes to cardiovascular activities on vacation, if you want to maximize your caloric output, you may choose higher-intensity (HIIT) ones that drive this more than lower-intensity (LIIS) ones. When it comes to cardio, the important thing to remember is to stay as active as possible. Remember, your planned exercise (EAT) contributes to your overall caloric output but it is only 5%. Your NEAT (Non-Exercise Activity Thermogenesis) contributes to 15% of your overall caloric threshold per day.

If you stay active during your vacation, you can potentially contribute more toward your overall caloric output on vacation than your planned cardio. Of course, it depends on what type of vacation you're taking. If you're going to an island and your plan is to lay out in the sunshine all day, your NEAT will probably be on the low end for the day. If that's the case, you'll want to rely more on your EAT to contribute as much of the 5% that you can toward your daily caloric output.

Conversely, if you're going to Europe, let's say, and you'll be walking most of your trip, you may want to consider doing only some resistance training to maintain your muscle volume since you'll be doing such a high level of NEAT that will be contributing to your overall caloric output. For a very active vacation that involves a lot of cardio and NEAT, caloric output becomes less of a concern (as long as your nutrition is on point), and resistance training takes priority for your planned exercise, to ensure you maintain your muscle. Regardless of what type of vacation you go on, a movement goal should be a priority that will ultimately contribute to your daily calorie output, contributing toward not exceeding your TDEE during vacation.

Successful Planning for Nutrition

On vacation, nutrition can sometimes be the hardest part of your fitness plan; however, successfully hitting your nutrition goals while traveling is certainly possible, especially with the ReShapeHER program. As discussed in previous chapters, the macronutrient you'll want to prioritize is protein. By prioritizing protein, you'll be able to support your lean muscle tissue while on vacation, as well as contribute toward your satiety. Carbohydrates and fats can be interchangeable in terms of how they are prioritized on vacation. Carbohydrates can often be easier to prioritize second, as they are easily accessible while traveling. Fats will be prioritized last in terms of your macronutrients. What will be critical however, is that you stay within your TDEE while you're away. As a reminder, should you over consume calories no matter what type of activities you've done, this will result in weight gain over time.

When it comes to traveling, making good choices on nutritious snacks with a great macronutrient profile is key. These choices can often set you up best for the day, as unnecessary calories consumed with snacks can often lead us to falling short of our fitness goals. For example, a 200-calorie protein bar (with 15 grams of protein, 25 grams of carbs, and eight grams of fat) would be a better choice than a 110-calorie bag of pretzels (with two grams of protein, 23 grams of carbohydrates, and one gram of fat). Although the pretzels are low in fat, they don't contain as much protein, which doesn't allow them to contribute as much not only to your daily protein requirements but also to your satiety, leaving you hungry for another snack that will also contribute to your TDEE. Personally, this is why I'm a huge proponent of bringing my own snacks, as much as possible, on vacation. I find that having these foods with me at the hotel room, poolside, and during many downtimes during a vacation helps me achieve my goals for each day and increases my satiety so I'm less likely to binge while going out. (Plus with the extra weight your snacks cost you in bringing them, you'll have that much weight to carry back souvenirs once the snacks are consumed!)

It is critical to choose snacks that have a good macronutrient profile like protein powder (I mix with water and may add powdered peanut butter), low-calorie protein chips, protein bars, veggies and peanut butter, trail mix, gluten-free oats with protein powder/peanut butter, etc. Oftentimes as mothers, since we always have snacks with us for the kids, we can end up consuming too much of them, resulting in us exceeding our daily TDEE. This is the area where understanding our snack macronutrients and being mindful with them through nutritional tracking, helps us maintain control even while we are on vacation.

While on vacation it is also important to be mindful of making the best choices for each of your three macronutrients and their ratios in the foods you are eating. (Note: You become better at this the more you track your foods on a consistent basis.) Lean pieces of chicken, red meat, and fish without unknown toppings and sauces are great choices for main entrees at restaurants and make great contributions toward your protein requirements.

Avoiding proteins that are fried helps to cut out unnecessary fats in your diet. For example, choosing grilled chicken versus fried, a fish fillet versus fish and chips, a pork chop versus carnitas fried in oil, a piece of steak versus chicken-fried steak, etc. can be excellent choices. Side dishes that include wholesome foods that are closest to their original and unadulterated form are the best choices for your carbohydrate requirements, including things like baked potatoes, rice, veggies, salads, etc. Higher fiber choices will not only allow for you to reach your daily fiber intake requirements (for women, this is a suggested 25g per day), but it will also help with your satiety.

As with proteins, avoiding fried side dishes always helps in avoiding unnecessary fats. So, choose a dry baked potato (limit the toppings by ordering them on the side and add sparingly), simple brown or white rice versus fried rice, a side of pasta with olive oil and salt versus a creamy sauce, whole pinto beans versus refried beans, etc.

With meals that have a carbohydrate as the centerpiece (as with pasta or rice dishes), I will often double my order of protein to contribute to my satiety and ensure that I'm hitting my protein requirements. Most of the time, you can fulfill your fat requirements simply by eating the foods that meet your protein and carbohydrate requirements, which is another reason why understanding the nutritional content of foods is so critical.

The area that most people need to be the most mindful of when eating out on vacation and away from their familiar foods is making good decisions about food preparation. Because it is the goal of a restaurant to make food taste good, this often means that more things are added to the foods to make them taste better. These condiments, additional sauces, dressings, etc. are usually heavy in fats and can quickly contribute to one's TDEE. This is why it's critical to understand if they are included in foods. You need to make the decision to have them placed on the side or simply avoid them altogether. Additionally, it makes it easier to track your foods if you're able to avoid a lot of these unknown additives, allowing you greater control over your fitness goals.

When eating out, one of the most important things you can understand and apply your knowledge, are with portion sizes. This is where many people fail in terms of their diet, especially when eating out, as it becomes harder to track serving sizes based on how food is plated. There are many techniques you can use to manage portion sizes while going out—using smaller dinnerware, asking for a half serving versus a whole, using your hands as a general guideline, etc.—but these are all generalizations in terms of what your unique portion sizes should be. If you haven't been able to track your macronutrients long enough to be able to eyeball your portion sizes, my best advice would be to consider your portion sizes by hand.

For example, a baseball (equivalent to the size of an average-sized fist) should measure about one cup. This is an appropriate portion size for raw or uncooked vegetables, whole fruit, or fruit juice. A tennis ball (equivalent to a small-scooped handful size) should measure about one half cup. This should be equal to a one-ounce equivalent for grains such as pasta, rice, oatmeal, etc. A thumb size measuring about one tablespoon should be an appropriate portion size for peanut butter, other nut spreads, etc. A postage stamp or the tip of the pointer finger to the first joint should measure about one teaspoon. This should be an appropriate size for oil, butter, and other types of fat. Regardless of the portion sizes for meals, it is critical that they are inclusive of your daily macronutrient requirements and fall within your TDEE to reach your ideal body composition.

Another way in which you can reach your fitness goals while eating out is to consume foods at restaurants that share their nutritional facts for the foods they serve. Due to a new law that was enacted on May 7, 2018 by the Federal Drug Administration, any restaurant or retail food establishment with more than 20 locations must provide customers with a calorie count on their food items. There are also many restaurants that voluntarily provide this information; however, many still do not. This is where it becomes critical to understand portion sizes so you can hit your nutritional goals as you track. It is also important to still be mindful of the many additional foods that end up on your plate such as sauces, bread, chips, etc. Even with given nutritional tracking values, it is important to exercise mindfulness when eating out as sometimes these values can provide you with a false sense of control as they are often not 100% accurate.

Alcohol

An additional key to making sure you stay on your fitness plan while eating out is to avoid foods or drinks that don't offer anything in terms of nutritional value. Alcohol, for example, can derail your fitness plan if consumed in large quantities or isn't consumed mindfully. There are many reasons why alcohol can keep you from obtaining your goals, but mainly it's because once consumed, your body focuses more on metabolizing alcohol instead of burning fat. Additionally, your body will burn the calories from the alcohol prior to fat stores, which doesn't allow for fat loss. Consuming alcohol also lowers your inhibitions and can make you feel hungrier, which can lead to overconsumption and a possible calorie surplus.

Although alcohol can negate our fitness efforts, there are ways to consume it mindfully and still reach your goals while on vacation. As I've mentioned in previous chapters, you can track alcohol intake into your macros by adding it to your fat or carbohydrate totals for the day. As you recall, alcohol is seven calories per gram, which is almost as many as a gram of fat (at nine calories per gram). If you plan to consume alcohol, you can simply track it into your macronutrient totals as a partial meal, consume fewer calories prior to consumption, or plan for it mindfully during the week to allow for higher calories per day but maintain your weekly average for your TDEE. Also, you can limit your alcohol consumption in terms of calories by choosing drinks that have a lesser amount of calories than others, such as a vodka soda (which boasts 64 calories for a one-ounce shot of vodka) instead of a mixed drink that may contain 3-4 times that amount.

When consuming alcohol and other non-nutritious drinks, you have to also be mindful of portion sizes, especially if they're not measured. Although restaurants may measure what they're pouring, when alcohol is consumed outside of a restaurant, especially on vacation, it's easy to over-consume as oftentimes as it may be poured straight from the bottle into the glass. Wine, for example (at five fluid ounces), is 123 calories. An average restaurant lists glasses of wine by eight-ounce portions, which contain a whopping 188 calories a glass. The calorie difference adds up. If you order a 750 ml bottle of wine from the menu, it will contain around 600 calories that are added to your dining experience. Mixers and other non-nutritional drinks such as sweetened juices and sodas can be tracked in a similar fashion; however, they would be tracked at four calories per gram as their base is sugar versus that of alcohol. However, keep in mind that these types of drinks, if very sweet, may contain many more calories than that of an alcoholic drink. One can of soda (12 fluid ounces) is equivalent to 150 calories, which is almost three times that of a one-ounce vodka with soda!

Reserving Calories With Your Daily or Weekly TDEE "Spread"

Sometimes, despite even your greatest efforts, ordering foods that are familiar in order to accomplish your nutritional tracking and fitness goals successfully isn't always realistic while on vacation. The way you can plan for the occasional meal out on vacation, is by creating a calorie reserve for that meal during the day/week, or by contributing more toward your caloric output (in terms of your EAT or NEAT). For example, you can choose to eat a lighter breakfast and/or lunch if you're having a meal that evening that you might not be able to track. (Personally, I try to reserve about 50% of my daily TDEE for meals like that.) Additionally, you can choose to do a longer workout (or maybe a more intense one) to make up for this calorie consumption toward your TDEE. Lastly, you can plan to have an active day that contributes more toward your NEAT to ensure that your possible caloric additions are accounted for.

In lieu of reserving calories over the day, thinking of your weekly TDEE and reserving calories for these types of meals on vacation, can often be most effective. If you go over your weekly calorie allotment for the day, you can simply deduct that consumption from your weekly goal and readjust your daily average again. Personally, I find that by doing this, I'm not so quick to feel guilty that I didn't hit my daily goals and I can still keep perspective for the rest of the week.

The Importance of Fiber

One of the most powerful things you can do to increase satiety with meals on vacation, and not add to a higher amount of calorie consumption, is increase the volume or fiber content of them. You can do this with fibrous foods that have lower calories, such as veggies. Lettuce is very low in calories yet can add a large amount of volume and fiber to any dish. Other veggies such as tomato, broccoli, cucumber, cauliflower, etc. are great choices to add to a meal. Be careful when ordering, however, as many veggies are served with butter in restaurants so be sure to ask for no butter or oil unless you are going to track these items (asking for them steamed is often the best way to order them). Additionally, side salads come with dressings that are too often extremely high in calories and fats. You can control not having these on your plate by ordering a low-cal or fat-free dressing instead, asking for dressings to be on the side and using them sparingly, or simply squeezing citrus juice (like a lime or lemon) over your lettuce for flavor.

Elevating Food Without Unnecessary Calories

One of the keys in avoiding unnecessary calories is to avoid all of the additives and condiments that we use in order to make our food taste good. Proper seasoning can go a long way in accomplishing this. You can make a piece of protein taste a hundred times better with the right amount and type of seasoning. Ordering things void of butter and asking for them to be blackened or heavily seasoned is a way to cut out unnecessary fat and/or calories in one's diet. Oftentimes, just a simple squeeze of citrus can elevate a dish versus feeling the need to drown it in a condiment.

Ultimately, practicing the ReShapeHER program can allow you to maintain your fitness goals while still enjoying vacationing. It requires some effort and mindfulness, but the benefit is knowing that you can control your fitness outcomes while still enjoying yourself on vacation. Should you fall off track during your vacation, the benefit of the ReShapeHER program is that you can quickly get back on track whenever you choose. In terms of a year, a few days or even a few weeks of being "off track" won't derail your long-term progress.

MAINTAINING YOUR RESHAPEHER BODY AFTER PREGNANCY

Pregnancy brought me to my biggest learning lesson I had with my overall fitness. It took me nine months to develop my precious miracle, and I couldn't expect my body to bounce back overnight. It would take time. This was a very humbling experience for me. I went from being a very strong, athletic woman to being winded just climbing up a small set of stairs. Although there is truth to the fact that the fitter you are prior to pregnancy, the quicker you will bounce back, this process still takes time. A mother has to adjust to the demands of taking care of a newborn while also trying to maintain her own fitness.

"Start Low and Go Slow"

Post-pregnancy for me required revisiting the basics when it came to my fitness. I had to learn how to "start low and go slow" once receiving clearance from my doctor. When it came to resistance training, I had to develop a new baseline, slowly building from that point. With cardio, I started with very low intensities and worked my way up to higher-intensity ones. When I didn't have the time or energy to do my EAT (planned exercise), I contributed the best I could to my NEAT, staying as active as possible during the day. This was often easy to accomplish after my second pregnancy because I had to run around after a toddler. I spent many hours doing NEAT while cleaning up around the house, pushing around the stroller, cooking and making baby food, etc. I did my best to make it to the gym to accomplish my EAT, but I gave myself a lot of grace when it came to allowing my body the time to heal and work its way back to the fitness level it was once at. I reminded myself that my overall movement contributions during the day were bringing me closer to my goal, despite whether or not I could find the time like I had before, to accomplish a planned workout.

Combatting Muscle Loss

I realized after having a long period of time with less movement than I had prior to pregnancy, as well as little protein consumption during this time (I craved foods that didn't have much), I lost a lot of muscle tissue. This loss of muscle tissue resulted in me having a less-than-ideal body composition, which I wasn't happy with. Additionally, my body felt weak as a result. This is the point at which many women try to diet down after pregnancy to achieve a better body composition. I knew this was not a successful approach. The only way I could achieve my ideal body composition was by practicing a solid fitness plan that allowed me to fulfill my nutritional requirements, build back the muscle I had lost and lose the body fat I had gained over pregnancy. After working with my healthcare provider to decide when I could successfully start the ReShapeHER program, I then entered a "maintenance" season for a while to set my baseline for my nutritional requirements and understand my true TDEE post-pregnancy. This was followed by an "off" season, in which I spent time building back my lean muscle tissue that had been lost during my pregnancy. My "off" season was then followed by an "on" season, in which I successfully lost a healthy amount of body fat. It was during my "on" season, that I realized how successful my practices had been, in that I was able to achieve a body composition that was superior to the one I had prior to pregnancy, and even compete in my first Bodybuilding show in my 40's and after having my second child!

Importance of Time and Patience

There is not a "one size fits all" when it comes to a specific period of time a mother can expect to achieve a desired body composition after pregnancy. As mothers, we must appreciate that it took the body nine months to endure the miraculous changes of creating a human being and it may certainly take this much time or more to return to the state it once was in. However, we need to trust that with a solid fitness plan (like the one outlined in the ReShapeHER program), our bodies after pregnancy have just as much of a chance to be fit after pregnancy than before. Sure, you may have some additional aesthetic scars or stretch marks, but your ability to obtain an amazing body composition is within your reach with the same basic principles as before.

In our modern-day society, a lot of pressures are placed on women to quickly return to a pre-baby state. With the presence of social media, these pressures are exacerbated with many celebrities showing off their post-baby bodies that seemingly lack any evidence of being postpartum. This leaves women with a sense of false expectation, and if these results aren't achieved with their own bodies, they may try to achieve them in unhealthy ways or give up their pursuit altogether. As a society, this is an area where we have failed women and mothers. Women are badasses. We are the only humans who can create life. I'm sure you would agree that we can create a kick-ass physique if we are given the right tools and support.

Being fit after pregnancy is absolutely possible when mothers are equipped with a solid foundation of fitness knowledge. The ReShapeHER program is based on a solid foundation of fitness knowledge that can be tailored to any mom, allowing her to achieve her fitness goals after pregnancy. My body is a testament to this plan. As a postpartum mom of two, I have been able to achieve a better body composition in my 40s than I had in my 20s and continue competing in Bodybuilding!

MAINTAINING INJURY PREVENTION WITH YOUR RESHAPEHER BODY

Similar to fitness after pregnancy, starting a fitness plan back up after injury will require a "start low and go slow" process, after getting clearance from your doctor, in addition to a greater amount of patience and time. Depending on how long you may have been injured for, your body may take as long, if not longer, to make a full recovery and bring you to the place that you once were before. You may need to make adjustments to your previous plan and achieve your fitness potential with modifications and work with your healthcare provider to determine when you can start with this program after experiencing an injury. However, the thing to remember is that **IT IS POSSIBLE.** With the ReShapeHER program, making attempts to avoiding injury or rebounding post-injury is absolutely possible, as it gives you the tools to maintain and/or grow your muscle tissue in order to achieve a better body composition after spending time with an injury.

Importance of Stretching, Warm-ups and Cool-downs

There are many things a mother can do to try and prevent injury. Daily stretching is a great way to do this. Taking the time to do 5-10 minutes of effective, full-body stretches can reduce stiffness and get the blood flowing. Additionally, taking the time to do a quick warm-up prior to a workout can be really effective. Warm-ups can include jumping jacks, a brisk walk on the treadmill, a quick ride on a bike, a few minutes on the stair stepper, etc (depending on your fitness level). Warming up is important, as it gradually revs up your cardiovascular system by raising your body temperature and increases blood flow to the muscles that will be trained. This may reduce muscle soreness and also possibly reduce the risk of injury. Along with warming up, cooling down allows for the gradual recovery of pre-exercise heart rate and blood pressure. It allows blood flow to be regulated after an intense workout.

Knowing Our Baseline

When starting a new fitness plan, it can be especially tempting to want to overestimate one's abilities. Oftentimes, without prior knowledge of a personal baseline and the ease of comparing ourselves to others, many mothers can get caught in this trap. It is important to understand that we are all on our own unique fitness journeys. As I've mentioned in a previous chapter, no two women can be compared when it comes to fitness. Comparisons are futile when it comes to nutritional requirements, body composition, tailored fitness plans, and so many other things. Basing one's abilities on the premise of comparing oneself to someone else's is a risk in itself, leading someone to possible injury.

It is critical that we all have a good understanding of where our baseline is and keep track of our progress along the way so that we don't overestimate what we can do and injure ourselves. This is especially important when as mothers, especially after pregnancy, our baselines will change from what they once were prior. Patience is key when it comes to making sure that you progress along a trajectory that is unique to you and your abilities. This is one of the reasons why the ReShapeHER program includes both a 3-Day Fitness Plan and a 5-Day Fitness Plan as it allows a mother to choose her starting fitness plan based on her fitness level. It allows a mother to "start low and go slow" in effectively building up her efforts, in order to gradually make progress in order to prevent injury.

"No Pain, No Gain" Doesn't Apply

When practicing a fitness plan, the old expression "no pain, no gain" shouldn't have to apply. This saying implies that pain has to be incurred for a good workout to have taken place, and this is simply not true. Understanding the difference between general pain and discomfort is key when it comes to avoiding injury in a fitness plan. Movements that induce pain should simply be stopped. Pain is the body's primary warning signal that alerts us to a problem. It may come on as pointed, shooting, sharp, aching, or irritating. It is meant to alert us that something is wrong. If we don't listen, we risk injury. Muscles can be activated and also grown without inducing pain or even soreness.

Discomfort, on the other hand, can indicate that our workouts have pushed us to improve, whether cardiovascularly or with our strength training. Discomfort can result in feelings such as muscle fatigue that can be experienced during workouts, such as the burning sensation of lifting a heavier weight, or with DOMS (delayed-onset muscle soreness) that occurs within one to two days after a weight lifting session. This can happen if you're new to a fitness plan, returning to a fitness routine after some time off, or doing more intense workouts. However, muscle soreness shouldn't be the goal and actually avoided if possible, as it could negate our future efforts. Progressing slowly during times of discomfort, whether that be during a workout or the ones following it, is critical to ensure that injury can be prevented. How pain and discomfort contrast is that a routine can be continued with discomfort but the same cannot be said of one that incurs pain. Understanding how to listen to the cues of pain and discomfort, and knowing what to do when they happen, is imperative in preventing injury with any fitness plan.

Benefits of Progressive Overload

Along with being mindful of pain and discomfort cues, the method of Progressive Overload that is incorporated in the ReShapeHER program is not only effective in developing stronger muscles over time but can also possibly prevent injury. As you conservatively increase the stress placed on the muscles beyond what they have initially dealt with, they will learn to adapt to the change of demands placed on them over time. This adaptation allows the body to be able to respond in order to avoid over training and thus prevent injury. The idea is that slowly exposing the muscle fibers to higher intensities, longer durations, and increased frequencies allows for them to effectively grow stronger and, therefore, prevent injury with this strength.

Importance of Rest

This can often be one of the hardest things to accomplish as a mother... getting rest. However, it is critical when practicing a fitness plan. During rest, our body repairs damaged tissues. Rest also replenishes our energy stores and adapts to the stress we've placed on it during exercise. If we don't rest, our body may become tired, therefore, becoming more susceptible to injury. And, as busy Moms, an injury is never easy to manage!

Importance of Good Technique

When it comes to any sport or fitness plan, ensuring that it is done with proper technique is also essential when it comes to avoiding unnecessary injuries. Proper technique is essential to ensure that the movements are done in the right way, targeting the appropriate muscle groups. When it comes to resistance training especially, a minor adjustment can mean a completely different muscle group (or multiple groups) can be engaged, whether this is planned or not. Engaging areas of the body or muscle groups that aren't warranted can easily lead to injury, especially if these areas are weak and at risk for taking on load that could lead to injury. For example, knowing how to perform a major compound lift like a deadlift is critical, otherwise the resulting injury could lead to a back injury. Because of the high risk of injury in this area, this can justify a reason to hire a coach or personal trainer to show you the proper ways in which to perform various exercises in your fitness plan. Once you know how to do this appropriately and effectively, you can then perform them with consistency and practice progressive overload over time.

How Nutrition Supports Injury Prevention

In order to try and prevent injury, a nutritious diet like the one incorporated into the ReShapeHER program is one of the greatest contributions a mother can make to her overall fitness efforts. As I've discussed in a previous chapter, the macronutrients and micronutrients consumed in our diets, and in their appropriate ratios, are what fuel our bodies in terms of energy and tissue growth. For example, without enough fats and especially carbohydrates, we wouldn't have the stamina to accomplish our workouts. Without enough protein, we wouldn't be fueling our bodies with the main macronutrient required for lean muscle tissue growth. Additionally, without the micronutrients these macronutrients provide, our bodies wouldn't be able to perform the number of functions we need in order to achieve our health and body composition goals.

This is one of the areas in which nutritional tracking and understanding one's macronutrient requirements is key in understanding how you can not only fuel and support your fitness efforts but also prevent injury. Additionally, staying hydrated is another key component to ensure that you are consuming the requirements that your body needs in order to work at optimum levels. A nutritious diet is not only important to avoid injury but also to heal from injury, as it can play a key role in controlling inflammation. Additionally, it provides key macronutrients and micronutrients for rebuilding injured tissue. Without key nutrients (protein, for example), muscle tissue cannot be supported and muscle atrophy could take place. It is important to understand this risk as it would minimize strength preservation and gain should it occur.

Hydration

Injury prevention can also be done by replacing water and electrolytes that are lost through sweat and physical activity. Water and electrolytes are essential in delivering nutrients that help our bodily tissues repair themselves when they're injured. Dehydration can cause muscle tension and a host of other things that can derail our fitness. Considering our bodies are made up of about 50-60% water, this should be enough for us to want to make sure we are contributing to the living oceans we are!

The difficult thing about injury is knowing when it is safe to return to exercising. This is where it is critical to work with a healthcare provider to determine when this should be. Patience must be exercised so that you heal and don't return too quickly and suffer a re-injury. Small steps are key when starting a routine back up, and you should closely listen to your body to ensure that you return when your body is able. Recovery from an injury can be successful with the right amount of time and patience. Once recovered, the ReShapeHER program can help you achieve your fitness goals with time and consistency.

MAINTAINING YOUR RESHAPEHER BODY WITH AN AUTOIMMUNE DISEASE

Living with an autoimmune disease is a difficult experience, especially when trying to accomplish your fitness goals. Symptoms such as difficulty sleeping, headaches, depression, fatigue, muscle pain, etc., are many of the things you may experience while trying to manage one. These symptoms, and others, make it more challenging to ensure that both nutritional and exercise goals are consistently met. It is critical that if you are living with an autoimmune disorder, that you understand how to listen to your body and take mindful steps to ensure that your overall health goals are being met with a solid fitness plan. It is also critical to work with a healthcare provider to make sure that your internal health is reflective of overall wellness.

The frustrating part of having an autoimmune disease is that many people will tell you that it's not possible to achieve your optimal goals in fitness while you manage one. This is BULLSHIT. It is possible to have an autoimmune disease and achieve your fitness goals as a postpartum mom. *I have been able to successfully manage my autoimmune thyroid disease I was diagnosed with 25 years ago (Hashimotos), as well as achieve my fitness goals.* Understanding how to do this takes time, patience and is highly individualized. The great thing about the ReShapeHER program, is that any mother can individualize it according to her health, lifestyle or fitness goals.

Stress and Autoimmune Diseases

Although people suffering from autoimmune diseases can have periods of being symptom-free, they can periodically have flare-ups that are often induced by stress. Chronic stress in the presence of an autoimmune disease can cause chronic inflammation, immune dysregulation, imbalances in gut health and many other issues in the body. Many factors can trigger a flare-up, including infections and other environmental factors. These are the reasons why when suffering from an autoimmune disease, stress management is vital.

Personally, this is an area that I find I have to carefully manage with Hashimotos Thyroiditis, in that stress plays a huge factor in my fitness abilities and outcomes. For example, in times of stress, I struggle with having the ability to resistance train at the capacity I should when practicing Progressive Overload, as my allostatic stress load is high. I end up scaling my frequency of resistance training back (as I'll often switch from the 5-Day ReShapeHER plan to the 3-Day one), in order to manage my stress. Also, stress can also induce a lot of inflammation for me, that causes me to adjust my daily movements. I will often scale back my resistance training and the intensity of my cardiovascular exercises, to reduce the inflammation I'm experiencing, allowing my body more time to recover. During times of stress, I pay close attention to my true body composition values, as it can be easy to get discouraged with the additional weight the scale reads when my body is inflamed. Through experience, I have been able to understand that this scale weight is temporary and I can keep my sanity by keeping a laser-focus on my body composition values, which ultimately, reveal my overall fitness progress.

Measuring Fitness Outcomes

Additionally, it becomes vital when trying to gauge overall fitness outcomes. When stress is induced and inflammation results, this can often affect the numbers we see on the scale when it comes to weight. This is the area that becomes the most discouraging for mothers suffering from autoimmune diseases, as they feel like their efforts aren't translating into results. For autoimmune sufferers, it becomes even more critical to remember that scale weight doesn't tell us the entire picture of our body composition. Mothers with autoimmune diseases need to be well versed in understanding their body composition versus relying on the scale to dictate their progress. When a mother is able to see that her muscle mass has either stayed the same or grown, her body fat hasn't increased and her water weight has increased, she can learn to stay the course when it comes to her fitness and understand that it is the result of inflammation versus body fat gain.

Exercise

Although healthy to practice, exercise is an activity that can induce stress, which is why it has to be more conservatively managed with sufferers of autoimmune disorders. Management includes more periods of rest and movements of lesser intensity and/or lower impact in order to prevent the stress that can result from regular exercise. Although exercise can induce stress, it can also provide sufferers of autoimmune disorders a boost of physical energy, production of endorphins that help with pain, alleviation of depression and/or anxiety, and possibly reducing inflammation that can occur as a result of the disorders.

When it comes to exercise, the ReShapeHER fitness plan can be tailored to a mother suffering with an autoimmune disease, in many ways, For example, with her EAT (planned exercise), she can choose the 3-Day

Fitness Plan over the 5-Day Fitness Plan, in order to achieve her goals but practice her fitness with a lesser amount of time during the week(s) that she may have less energy. She will be able to take advantage of her NEAT (unplanned exercise), that she could swap for her EAT, and achieve her daily steps that will contribute 15% to her overall TDEE (as discussed in previous chapters). She can apply the principles to Progressive Overload according to her own efforts and advance when she has the energy to do so. With all of these benefits, it is critical for a mother to work with her healthcare provider to understand how she can tailor these programs to her needs.

Diet

When it comes to inflammation, a healthy diet that ensures that you aren't making a further contribution to this inflammation is essential in addition to practice. Ensuring that a diet consists of lots of fruits and vegetables, incorporating enough Omega 3 fatty acids into your diet, and drinking plenty of fluids is key. Foods such as processed meats, sugar, flour, fried foods, alcohol, etc. are typically what you want to steer clear from to avoid a rise in inflammation and associated symptoms.

Nutrition becomes difficult when managing an autoimmune disease, as sufferers tend to crave higher carbohydrate and sugary foods that cause inflammation, due to fatigue. The additives in these foods can also contribute to the "feel-good" serotonin boost when suffering from anxiety or depression as a result of an autoimmune disorder. Alcohol can often be difficult to avoid, as it has the ability to temporarily numb any pain and combat anxiety or depression that results from an autoimmune disease. Dieting or being in a state of a caloric deficit can add stress to the body, especially when done aggressively. For sufferers of autoimmune diseases, this added stress can contribute to further inflammation. Therefore, those with autoimmune diseases may benefit from having more days in a "maintenance" season to break up days of dieting efforts.

As part of her nutrition, a mother with an autoimmune disease will also need to be careful what she consumes in terms of her liquids in addition to her foods. Fatigue and low energy can be the culprit for a mother with an autoimmune disease to grab sugary sodas and drinks that are high in caffeine to keep her energy levels up, which may also contribute to inflammation. It is critical that mothers are aware of these types of patterns not only with their foods but also with their drinks, when it comes to managing their overall stress and inflammation.

Along with a mother being able to tailor her exercise efforts to achieve her goal as an autoimmune sufferer, she can also tailor her diet to her goals with the ReShapeHER program. This program allows a mother to tailor her nutritional efforts to reach her goals, despite her circumstances. Through her individual TDEE and macronutrient values, as well as her experience with nutritional tracking she'll obtain through this program, a mother will be able to fulfill her nutritional requirements, allowing her body to have the best chance at combating inflammation. Through this process, she'll be able to understand what foods serve her body the best or what foods cause her to experience symptoms. She'll also be able to make changes in a conservative manner when it comes to her seasons, making small adjustments over time that don't induce stress and inflammation, bringing her closer to her health and fitness goals.

Rest and Recovery

Mothers suffering from autoimmune issues, will need to ensure that they are getting plenty of rest each day. Prioritizing sleep is critical, as it also helps to reduce stress and inflammation. For mothers, getting a minimum of seven hours of sleep a night and taking time to recover from their workouts, is key to maintaining low inflammation. They will need to take more time to listen to their bodies and take the time to rest more often, if need be. Patience becomes a virtue when a mother is doing her best to practice rest and also work to achieve her fitness goals but it can be done effectively with the ReShapeHER program.

Journaling

When gauging progress for an autoimmune sufferer, it can be incredibly helpful to keep a journal of daily activities and nutrition. This would include both your planned exercise (EAT) and unplanned (NEAT). Journaling about foods that you ate and possibly side effects to them, are also helpful. Tracking emotions and feelings are another good way to gauge whether or not positive or negative patterns are being developed and making the necessary changes as needed over time. Using an app (like the MyFitnessPal one I mentioned in previous chapters), allows you to not only track your TDEE and macronutrients as foods are consumed, but also have a note section that allows you to journal your movements you are making and the foods you are consuming to reach your fitness goals.

When you have an autoimmune disease as a mother, this shouldn't preclude you from achieving your fitness goals. Although it takes some additional considerations to accomplish them, all of these things can be supported with the ReShapeHER program. By practicing this program with consistency and time, you can learn to "trust the process," knowing that regardless of your pace, you will ultimately reach your fitness goal.

NOTES

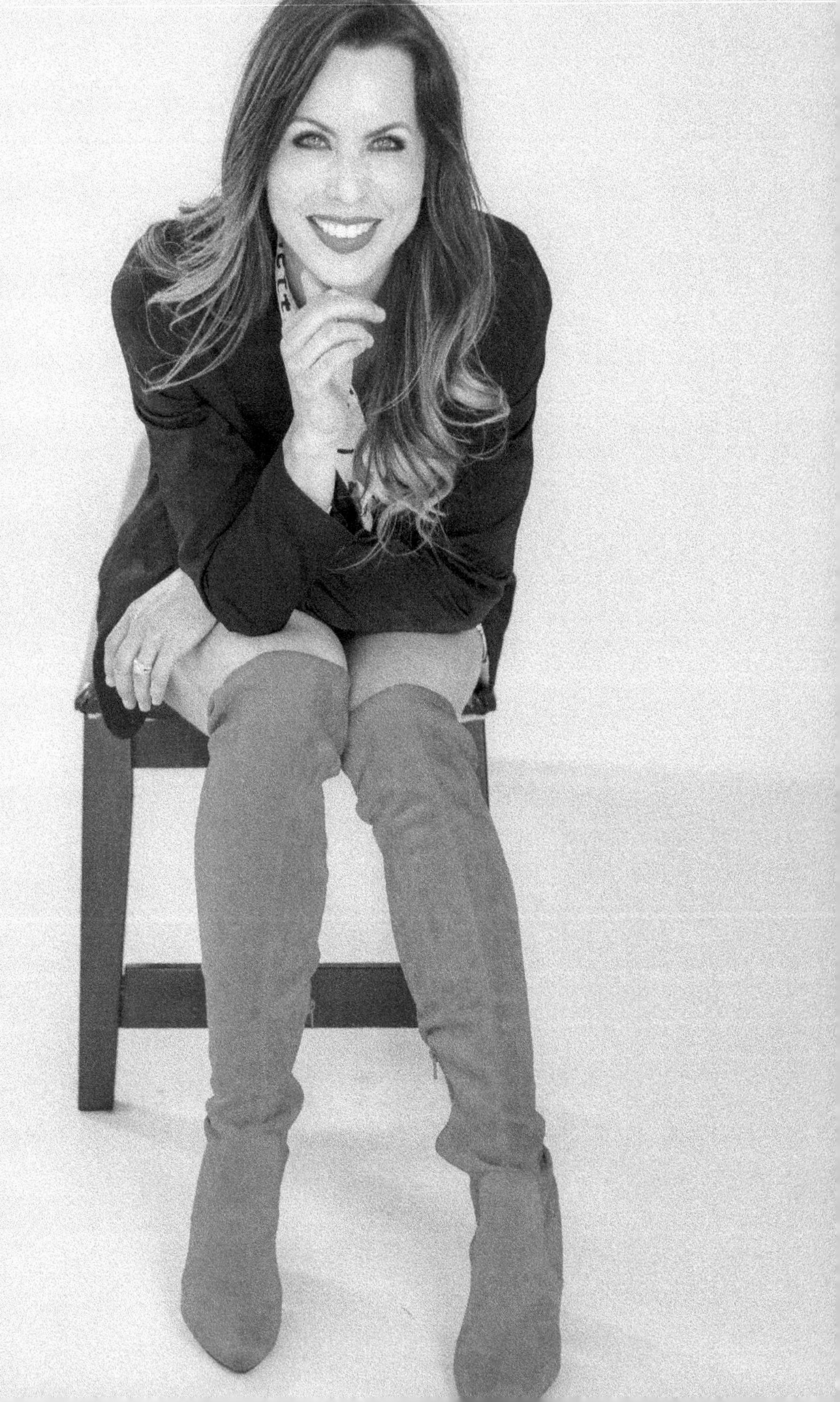

14

My Top 10 ReShapeHER Fitness Lessons

THIS BOOK WOULDN'T BE COMPLETE without me sharing these invaluable lessons with you, my fellow mother, as you commit to taking the time to work on achieving your greatest fitness potential! Please read through them all, as they are not mentioned in any particular order. They say that life's lessons are a beautiful gift, but they don't always come wrapped up in sparkling wrapping paper and shiny bows. Often these lessons involve tragedy, but in this, we gain wisdom. Sometimes these lessons bring joy. . . we bask in those. Other times, we learn lessons when we've least expected to, just like amazing memories on a trip that involves no itinerary. This is not the way I choose to travel, but then again, there is very little I can control about this amazing thing called life and the lessons it brings. What I can control, however, is how I share these invaluable lessons. And, I couldn't think of a better way to do this, than with another amazing mother like yourself.

LESSON #1:

We are ALL insecure

Sometimes we like to think that other Moms have it all together when it comes to life. Truth is, we don't. Some of us are just better at hiding our shortcomings and insecurities than others. Some of the fittest and most beautiful people I've ever met were also the most insecure. So, if you're ever feeling like you've gained a few pounds and you're feeling like everyone will notice, chances are, they won't. Most people are so caught up in their own heads to worry about noticing those details in others.

LESSON #2:

Consistency is KEY

One of the greatest things keeping most mothers from achieving their goals, doesn't lie in the fancy details of a nutrition or training program, but rather in the consistency of repeating the basic principles that equate to a fit and healthy lifestyle. If we spent more time doing the simple things and doing them well, we would have so much more success. Too often, we get caught up in the details. If you apply the basic principles of the ReShapeHER program to your life, you WILL see fitness results over time!

LESSON #3:

ANY MOVEMENT, small or large, leads us to our GOALS

Oftentimes as mothers, we get discouraged when we aren't able to make the advancements that we once hoped, towards our health and fitness goals. We overlook connecting the dots on smaller advancements, and instead, sometimes give up entirely if we can't make larger ones. We put timelines on things, and when these timelines aren't met, we stop pursuing our goals. We need to remember that small steps eventually add up and can lead us to our goals. When it comes to our fitness, all of our little successes add up to eventually lead us to something that we've always dreamed of! The important thing is that we stay the course.

LESSON #4:

Your MIND holds your greatest potential

Simply put, what you think you can achieve, is what you will. As mothers, we have to believe in ourselves and our capabilities. If we don't, our mind will become the antagonist to our goals and our bodies will follow suit. If you BELIEVE you can have the body composition you desire, YOU WILL achieve it!

LESSON #5:

Growth doesn't happen in your "COMFORT ZONE"

Just like we need to challenge our muscles to grow, we need to challenge ourselves to live outside our comfort levels from time to time. It is in this space that magic happens. Risk doing something you might hate... at least after doing it, you'll know. But on the flip side, if you love it, you'll be happy you took the plunge to try it! If you feel uncomfortable doing something you know you should be doing, chances are, you're in a growth stage.

LESSON #6:

You can't change your genetics, but you can affect them with LIFESTYLE and BEHAVIORAL modifications

When it comes to fitness, every mother can make amazing improvements to their body type with a solid fitness plan, regardless of their starting point! This is the reason why I am confident the ReShapeHER Program will bring you these amazing results if you practice it consistently!

LESSON #7:

AGE is just a NUMBER

I've met mothers who are much younger than me, that aren't healthy or fit due to their lifestyles, and they've aged quickly. I've also met mothers who are much older than myself, that are incredibly fit and could easily pass for being 10-20 years younger than they are. This is where age is just a number, as our overall wellness dictates our longevity. Focus on what matters and not the number! I am proof that you can be the fittest you've ever been after having kids and also at an older age!

LESSON #8:

You are what you EAT

You can't overlook science when it comes to what you feed your body. If you don't give it the proper fuel to support your goals, they can't be reached. What you eat matters! This is the reason why nutritional education is a large part of the ReShapeHER Program

LESSON #9:

When mothers SUPPORT one another, INCREDIBLE THINGS HAPPEN

There is no greater force than a tribe of mothers that support one another and adjust each other's crowns. When we realize how powerful we are together, and our collective contribution to raising the future, we can begin to comprehend how important this is. As mothers, we can positively change the world, by sharing our knowledge, life lessons and love with one another. When we support one another with our fitness journeys, there is room for us all to reach our goals. It is my hope that we all take heed to this power and use it to create a place for all of us mothers in the Fitness world.

LESSON #10:

NEVER STOP LEARNING

Through the process of learning we improve... our outlook, our beliefs and our abilities. By keeping our intellectual curiosity alive, we are able to capture all of the valuable lessons that our fitness journey has to offer and be able to share them with others. And the great thing about this is that life never stops teaching!

Endnotes

1 National Center for Chronic Disease Prevention and Health Promotion
CDC Health Schools
https://www.cdc.gov/healthyschools/obesity/index.htm#:~:text=In%20the%20United%20States%2C%20the,than%20tripled%20since%20the%201970s.&text=In%202017%E2%80%932018%2C%20about%201,%2D19%20year%20olds

2 Fryar CD, Carroll MD, Afful J. Prevalence of overweight, obesity, and severe obesity among children and adolescents aged 2–19 years: United States, 1963–1965 through 2017–2018. NCHS Health E-Stats. 2020.
https://www.cdc.gov/nchs/data/hestat/obesity-child-17-18/overweight-obesity-child-H.pdf

3 National Center for Health Statistics
Prevention of Obesity Among Adults and Youth: U.S, 2015-2016
Craig M. Hales, M.D., Margaret D. Carroll, M.S.P.H., Cheryl D. Fryar, M.S.P.H., and Cynthia L. Ogden, Ph.D.
https://www.cdc.gov/nchs/products/databriefs/db288.htm#:~:text=The%20prevalence%20of%20obesity%20among%20U.S.%20youth%20was%2018.5%25%20in,5%20years)

4 National Library of Medicine
Recommended Dietary Allowances, 10th ed
https://www.ncbi.nlm.nih.gov/books/NBK234922/

5 Health Benefits of Dietary Fiber
First published: 25 March 2009
James W Anderson, Pat Baird, Richard H Davis Jr, Stefanie Ferreri, Mary Knudtson, Ashraf Koraym, Valerie Waters, Christine L Williams
https://doi.org/10.1111/j.1753-4887.2009.00189.x

6 National Institute of Health (NIH)
Advanced Nutrition v.9 (3); May 2018
https://www.ncbi.nlm.nih.gov/pmc/articles/PMC5952928/

7 National Institute of Health (NIH)
Advanced Nutrition; v.5(6); Nov 2014
https://www.ncbi.nlm.nih.gov/pmc/articles/PMC4224210/

8 National Institute of Health (NIH)
PubMed - Nutrients 2021 Jan; 13(1); 143
https://www.ncbi.nlm.nih.gov/pmc/articles/PMC7824178/

9 Ibid

10 World Health Organization
WHO updates guidelines on Fats and Carbohydrates; July 17 2023
https://www.who.int/news/item/17-07-2023-who-updates-guidelines-on-fats-and-carbohydrates

11 National Institute of Health (NIH)
Do trans fatty acids from industrially produced sources and from natural sources have the same effect on Cardiovascular disease risk factors in health subjects? Results of the Trans Fatty Acids Collaboration {TRANSFACT} studyAM J Clin Nutr March 2008, vol. 87, no.3
https://pubmed.ncbi.nlm.nih.gov/18326592/

12 World Health Organization
WHO updates guidelines on Fats and Carbohydrates; July 17 2023
https://www.who.int/news/item/17-07-2023-who-updates-guidelines-on-fats-and-carbohydrates

13 Bone Health and Osteoporosis Foundation: Sept 28, 2016, https://americanbonehealth.org/fracture/fracture-risk-factors/#:~:text=Women%20are%20far%20more%20likely,-less%20dense%20than%20men's%20bones/

14 Women's Health Magazine: "Why Some People Are So Prone to Yo-Yo Dieting", K. Aleisha Fetters, Sept 6, 2016, https://www.womenshealthmag.com/weight-loss/a19896749/why-do-people-yo-yo-diet/

15 Journal of Medical Internet Research: Vol 22, No. 10; Feb 13, 2020, Charlotte Evenepoel, BSc, MSc; Egbert Cleavers, BSc, MSc, PhD; Lise DeRoover, BSc, MSc, PhD; Wendy VanLoo, BA; Christophe Matthys BSc MSc, PhD; Kristine Verbeke,BSc, MSc, PhD
https://www.jmir.org/2020/10/e18237/

16 Journal of Medical Internet Research: Vol 22, No. 10; Feb 13, 2020, Charlotte Evenepoel, BSc, MSc; Egbert Cleavers, BSc, MSc, PhD; Lise DeRoover, BSc, MSc, PhD; Wendy VanLoo, BA; Christophe Matthys BSc MSc, PhD; Kristine Verbeke,BSc, MSc, PhD
https://www.jmir.org/2020/10/e18237/

17 Medscape: https://reference.medscape.com/calculator/846/mifflin-st-jeor-equation

18 National Institute of Health (NIH) Sports Medicine 2021; 51(Suppl 1): 43–57; PMCID: PMC8566643; https://www.ncbi.nlm.nih.gov/pmc/articles/PMC8566643/#:~:text=Currently%2C%20the%20American%20College%20of,the%20primary%20focus%20%5B82%5D

19 Health.com - 8 Protein Deficiency Symptoms; September 25, 2023; Jilian Kubala, RD.; https://www.health.com/nutrition/signs-not-eating-enough-protein

20 National Institute of Health (NIH), Pub Med - Adv Nutrition; v.5(6); 2014 Nov; PMC4224210, https://www.ncbi.nlm.nih.gov/pmc/articles/PMC4224210/

21 National Institute of Health (NIH); Pub Med - Br J Sports Med; 2019 Nov;53(22):1393-1396. doi: 10.1136/bjsports-2018-099420. Epub 2018 Aug 14;
https://pubmed.ncbi.nlm.nih.gov/30108061/

22 My Fitness Pal application; https://www.myfitnesspal.com/

23 Ibid

24 Legion Athletics: How Long Does It Take To Build Muscle? Michael Matthews (rev. by Brian Grant, M.D.) https://legionathletics.com/how-long-does-it-take-to-build-muscle/

25 National Institutes of Health (NIH) Pub Med; Muscle Size Responses to Strength Training in Young and Older Men and Women; JAm Geriatr Soc; 2001 Nov;49(11):1428-33. doi: 10.1046/j.1532-5415.2001.4911233.x. https://pubmed.ncbi.nlm.nih.gov/11890579/

26 Bodybuilding.com: Building the Mind-Muscle Connection; Jake Stewart, May 5, 2023
https://www.bodybuilding.com/content/building-the-mind-muscle-connection.html

27 Amercian Council of Exercise (ACE) How Many Reps Should You Be Doing? Pete McCall, March 11, 2016; https://www.acefitness.org/resources/everyone/blog/5867/how-many-reps-should-you-be-doing/

28 American Council of Exercise (ACE) Weight Lifting Tempo & Amp; Sets: How To Select the Right Sets For Your Clients; July 3, 2014; https://www.acefitness.org/resources/pros/expert-articles/4931/weight-lifting-tempo-amp-sets-how-to-select-the-right-sets-for-your-clients/

29 Amercian Council of Exercise (ACE) How Many Reps Should You Be Doing? Pete McCall, March 11, 2016; https://www.acefitness.org/resources/everyone/blog/5867/how-many-reps-should-you-be-doing/

30 American College of Sports Medicine Guidelines for Resistance Training for Health and Fitness - brochure; Michael R. Esco, Ph.D., HFS, CSCS*D, product of ACSM's Consumer Information Committee.
https://www.prescriptiontogetactive.com/static/pdfs/resistance-training-ACSM.pdf

31 Amercian Council of Exercise (ACE) How Many Reps Should You Be Doing? Pete McCall, March 11, 2016; https://www.acefitness.org/resources/everyone/blog/5867/how-many-reps-should-you-be-doing/

32 National Institute of Health (NIH) PubMed; Mayo Clin Proc; v. 87 (6); 2012 Jun; PMC3538475 v.87(6); 2012 Jun. https://www.ncbi.nlm.nih.gov/pmc/articles/PMC3538475

33 Center for Disease Control (CDC) Guidelines - How Much Activity Do Adults Need? June 2022; usa.gov. https://www.cdc.gov/physicalactivity/basics/adults/index.htm

34 National Institute of Health (NIH) Higher Daily Step Count Linked With Lower All-cause Mortality; March 24, 2020 https://www.nih.gov/news-events/news-releases/higher-daily-step-count-linked-lower-all-cause-mortality

35 CNET, Lisa Eadicicco; Jan 29 2022 https://www.cnet.com/tech/mobile/fitness-trackers-are-getting-more-personal-powerful-in-2022-and-beyond/

36 National Strength and Conditioning Association by NSCA's Essentials of Personal Training, Second Edition; May 2017: https://www.nsca.com/education/articles/kinetic-select/determination-of-resistance-training-frequency

37 American College of Sports Medicine Guidelines for Resistance Training for Health and Fitness - brochure, Michael R. Esco, Ph.D., HFS, CSCS*D, product of ACSM's Consumer Information Committee. https://www.prescriptiontogetactive.com/static/pdfs/resistance-training-ACSM.pdf

38 National Academy of Sports Medicine (NASM) Progressive Overload Explained: Grow Muscle and Strength Today, Andre Adams, 2022, https://blog.nasm.org/progressive-overload-explained#:~:text=When%Should%20You%20Progressively%20Overload,progressions%20every%202%2D4%20weeks

39 Ibid

40 American College of Sports Medicine Guidelines for Resistance Training for Health and Fitness - brochure, Michael R. Esco, Ph.D., HFS, CSCS*D, product of ACSM's Consumer Information Committee. https://www.prescriptiontogetactive.com/static/pdfs/resistance-training-ACSM.pdf

41 Ibid

42 National Strength and Conditioning Association by NSCA's Essentials of Personal Training, Second Edition; May 2017: https://www.nsca.com/education/articles/kinetic-select/determination-of-resistance-training-frequency

43 Center for Disease Control (CDC) How Much Physical Activity Do Adults Need? https://www.cdc.gov/physical-activity-basics/guidelines/adults.html?CDC_AAref_Val=

44 American Heart Association (AHA) Strength and Resistance Training Exercise: https://www.heart.org/en/healthy-living/fitness/fitness-basics/strength-and-resistance-training-exercise

45 National Institute of Health (NIH) PubMed; Effect of Reduced Training Frequency on Muscular Strength Int. Journal of Sports Med; J.E. Graves 1988 Oct;9(5):316-9. doi: 10.1055/s-2007-1025031, PMID: 3246465; DOI: 10.1055/s-2007-1025031 https://pubmed.ncbi.nlm.nih.gov/3246465/

46 Body Cardio – What are the normal ranges for body composition?" https://support.withings.com/hc/en-us/articles/220035767-Body-Cardio-What-are-the-normal-ranges-for-body-composition

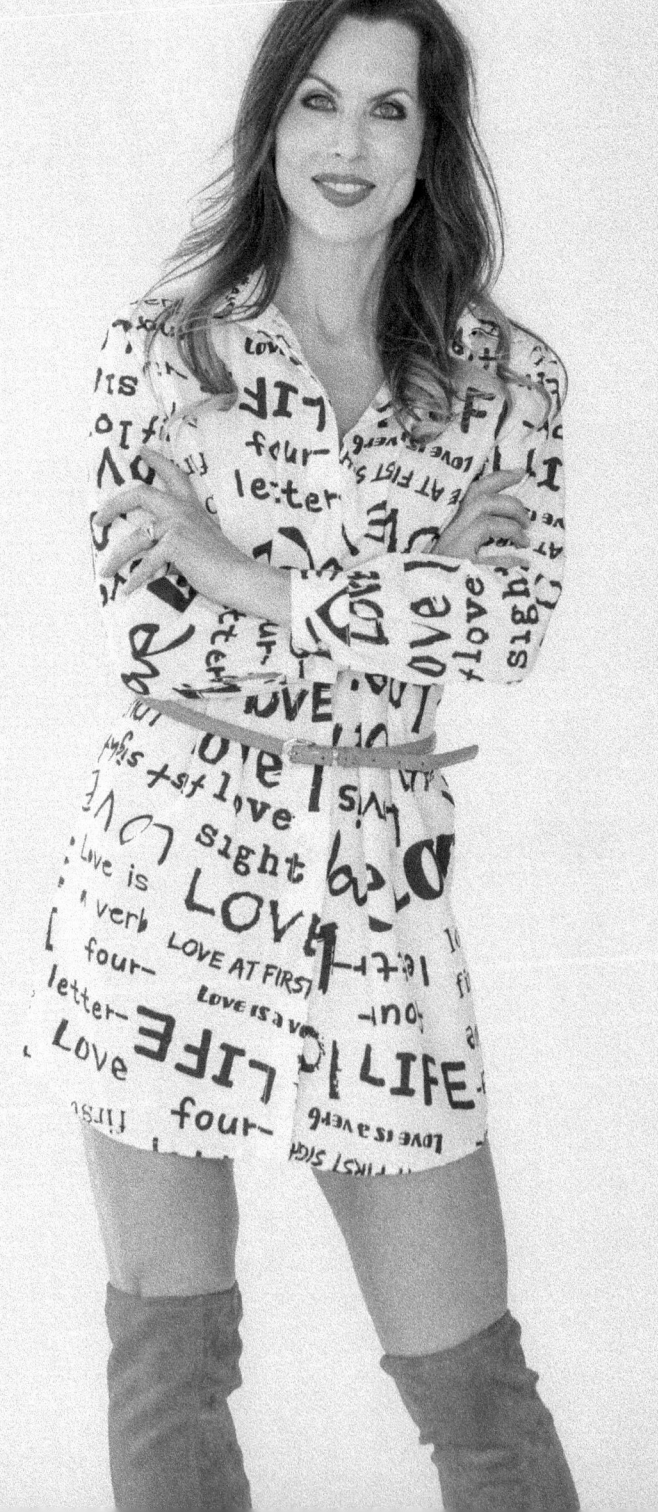
LIFE
four-
letter
LOVE
love
sight
Love is
LOVE
LOVE AT FIRST
letter-
Love
LIFE
four-

About the Author

AUTHOR CASSIE MORELL is a NCCPT Certified Coach and Personal Trainer through ISSA, a certified Precision Nutrition coach and has earned a degree in Biology from Chapman University. As an alumni collegiate athlete and nationally qualified Master Bodybuilding competitor, she is able to speak to nutrition and fitness principles that bring results to a female body.

Cassie understands what it's like to be a busy Mom that is motivated to achieve her fitness goals with limited time. She is dedicated to helping fellow moms save TIME and MONEY, as she teaches them how they can quickly achieve and maintain their ideal body composition goals with the ReShapeHER Program she has developed. This book, as well as the ReShapeHER Program, both serve to fulfill Cassie's true "calling" in her life...to help carve a place in the Fitness industry for mothers. She wants to help fill the void of nutritional and fitness education that doesn't serve our mothers in society and combat the falsifications and misinformation that keep them from reaching their fitness goals. Her passion is fueled by her own experience, being raised by a single mother that struggled to reach her goals, without the support she could've had with this type of education.

Cassie balances her career along with being a wife and mother to two young kids that are also athletes and have busy schedules of their own. One of her greatest supporters is her husband whom she considers her best friend. She is also an avid traveler, as she carves out time to cross the globe from Los Angeles with her family, as she enjoys visiting new places and embracing different cultures that allow her to continue learning and evolving. She enjoys living "outside" of her comfort zone, as she knows that this is the area in which she's able to grow. Like her Zodiac sign, she's a true Libra at heart, doing her best to find balance in all things, including her pursuit in coming up with the healthiest dessert recipes to satisfy her sweet tooth while also reaching her nutritional goals. As the oldest of three sisters and having a driven and ambitious personality, Cassie's is reflective of her brand...BOLD, HONEST and AUTHENTIC. She values people, places and brands that reflect this same type of sincerity and transparency.

From understanding how to start your fitness journey off with self-love to maintaining it with a solid fitness plan like the ReShapeHER Program highlighted in this book, Cassie speaks directly to the psyche of a mother in helping her understand more about herself and also her fitness potential. She helps mothers navigate the muddied waters of the fitness industry, guiding them with solutions based on scientific principles, and showing them how they can get results in as little as 12 weeks. Her ReShapeHER Program is straightforward, easy to follow and allows mothers to achieve and maintain a long-lasting, healthy body composition.

Through this book and her ReShapeHER Program, Cassie hopes to collectively raise the status of mothers through fitness education, awareness, and literacy. She expresses in her work that is time for us to show ourselves how to RESET our dysfunctional thought processes when it comes to fitness, time for us to REFRAME the way we think about what is possible when it comes to our fitness potential and time to optimally RESHAPE our bodies by consistently practicing successful fitness habits that contribute to us reaching and maintaining our best overall health as moms. Like she says in her book, "There's no better time than now!"

CASSIE MORELL

www.CassieMorell.com

www.ingramcontent.com/pod-product-compliance
Lightning Source LLC
Chambersburg PA
CBHW052127030426
42337CB00028B/5055
9798990931817